"Beautiful, brave, and heartbreaking, *A Womb in the Shape of a Heart* illuminates both the joys of motherhood and the grief of miscarriage in equal measure. With suspenseful storytelling and honest revelation, this is a compelling read."

-Beth Powning, author of *Shadow Child: An Apprenticeship in Love and Loss*

"This book is a love letter: to the cherished babies the author has lost, to her cherished son who stayed, to her loving husband, to the health-care professionals who guided them through with kindness, and also to herself—the person she was before, during, and after her miscarriages. It is also a love letter to anyone who has ever experienced the everlasting ache of pregnancy loss. Gallant has opened up a space for us where grief and joy can exist together. Her tender words burrowed into me and found a home, and I'm so grateful she wrote them."

-Jessica Westhead, author of *Worry*

"Gallant's exquisite chronicle of loss transforms the private anguish of so many women into revelatory beauty. Candid, fierce, and embracing, this is a lyric testimony to the ways hope can both betray and redeem us…an elegy filled with wisdom and grace."

-Lorri Neilsen Glenn, award-winning author of *Following the River: Traces of Red River Women*

"Becoming a mother is emotional and uncharted territory no matter what our outcomes. Gallant's deeply resonant memoir is both raw and gentle, a kindness for those of us who have found grief and tumult as well as hope, resilience, and renewal along that journey."

-Kate Inglis, award-winning author of *Notes for the Everlost: A Field Guide to Grief*

"Many mothers—people with children as well as those who long for them—will be grateful that Joanne Gallant has shared her story. I know I am. Her debut memoir contains so many of the paradoxes of life: how the greatest joys can be underscored with the deepest terrors, how hope can be so tightly woven into grief, but ultimately, it is the love in this book that will stay with me. Her love for her child, for her husband, for the babies she lost, but also for the vulnerability she reveals in this moving book, which, in another one of those paradoxes, she shows us can also be an act of love."

-Harriet Alida Lye, author of *The Honey Farm* **and** *Natural Killer*

"*A Womb in the Shape of a Heart* is a must-read for anyone who knows the heartache of pregnancy loss. I wish this book existed when I was going through my own experience with infertility and multiple miscarriages. Joanne's candid memoir is honest, hopeful, and soothing."

-Ariel Ng Bourbonnais, author of *Through, Not Around*

Printed and bound in Canada
NB1563

Cover artwork © Briana Corr Scott

Editor: Whitney Moran
Design: Rudi Tusek

Library and Archives Canada Cataloguing in Publication

Title: A womb in the shape of a heart : my story of miscarriage and
   motherhood / Joanne Gallant.
Names: Gallant, Joanne, author.
Identifiers: Canadiana (print) 20210215100 | Canadiana (ebook) 20210215275 |
   ISBN 9781771089760 (softcover) | ISBN 9781771089838 (EPUB)
Subjects: LCSH: Gallant, Joanne. | LCSH: Gallant, Joanne—Health. | LCSH:
   Miscarriage—Patients—Canada—Biography. | LCSH: Infertility, Female—
   Patients—Canada—Biography. | LCSH: Motherhood. | LCSH: Postpartum
   depression—Patients—Canada—Biography. | LCGFT: Autobiographies.
Classification: LCC RG648 .G35 2021 | DDC 618.3/920092—dc23

 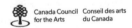 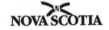

Nimbus Publishing acknowledges the financial support for its publishing activities from the Government of Canada, the Canada Council for the Arts, and from the Province of Nova Scotia. We are pleased to work in partnership with the Province of Nova Scotia to develop and promote our creative industries for the benefit of all Nova Scotians.

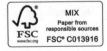

A WOMB IN THE SHAPE OF A HEART

My Story of Miscarriage and Motherhood

Joanne Gallant

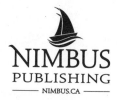

NIMBUS
PUBLISHING
— NIMBUS.CA —

For Teddy and Joey

"I'm a mother.
I'm a mother tossed in the wave of my love;
helpless, vulnerable.
I'm a mother, whether my son is here or not,
whether my son is alive or not."

–Beth Powning, *Shadow Child*

Author's Note

This is a work of non-fiction. However, in some cases, names of individuals have been altered to protect their privacy. Some characters have been amalgamated into singular entities for the purpose of narrative.

1

▼

BEFORE I EVEN TAKE THE TEST, I KNOW IT IS GOING TO BE
positive.

I am standing in my bathroom, waiting impatiently for the
three minutes to pass so I can hold tangible proof of what I already
know: I am pregnant. I look at my reflection in the mirror above
the sink and I run my hands over my stomach, convinced I see
a slight bulge that wasn't there before. I feel as changed now as
the time I lost my virginity to my high school boyfriend and I
was certain everyone could read it on my face.

The alarm dings on my phone, which is sitting precariously
on the edge of the bathroom sink, and I pick up the test I peed
on. It's unmistakable: two pink lines. I clutch the test tightly,
giving myself a brief moment alone with the child I already love.

Joey looks up when I walk into the next room, his brown eyes
so familiar, and hope fills the space between us.

"I'm pregnant," I say, smiling. And just like that, our first baby
is born into reality.

This pregnancy will result in the birth of a baby after nine
months, a fact I learned in the earliest of sexual-health classes as a
child. The days when we all giggled at the words *penis* and *vulva*,
and our teacher allowed us a moment of laughter before clapping
her hands together and saying sharply, *Enough!* Infertility was
not taught in school. As a newly pregnant woman, and even as a
nurse, I would not have been able to explain all the ways in which
a pregnancy can go wrong. My own fertility was an assumption
that had never before been challenged, and I was following the
script of a life I had always believed would be mine.

I do what most women do when they are newly pregnant. I keep my early condition a secret, knowing you wait twelve weeks before you deliver the news in the rare case your pregnancy ends before then. Even the word *miscarriage* would have felt foreign leaving my mouth—like the time I tried to learn Mandarin during a brief trip to Hong Kong in my twenties and I asked the waiter for more rice but was shown the door to the bathroom instead.

I learn an entirely new language during my path to motherhood, and I spend those early days of pregnancy searching and re-searching the symptoms I am experiencing. I am exhausted, falling asleep before nine each night, and my bloated abdomen ripples with pains reminding me of menstrual cramps. I create a Pinterest board of nursery-theme ideas and I buy a tiny onesie that I cradle whenever I am alone, imagining the baby that will one day wear it. Those three weeks of pregnancy are filled with the naïve certainty that this child will be born.

I am at work one afternoon, not long after holding that positive pregnancy test, when I suddenly buckle over in pain. I excuse myself to the bathroom, where I see a menacing swirl of blood pooling in the toilet beneath me. Bleeding at seven weeks pregnant had not come up in of any of the research I had done on early pregnancy. I stand and pace in the small bathroom, hoping I am mistaken. Maybe I'm not bleeding after all. Maybe if I close my eyes the blood will go away. Yet, every time I look, the dark red is still there. My heart rate quickens, my hands go numb as my body fills with dread. I leave my nursing shift abruptly, feeling guilty for abandoning the now short-staffed unit, and I spend hours waiting in a busy emergency department.

Joey is sitting beside me on the uncomfortable waiting-room chairs. They are slick blue vinyl with unnaturally straight backs, likely designed with much shorter wait times in mind, and I sit with my legs crossed, as if by squeezing my thighs tightly together I can stop a miscarriage from happening. When I finally see the doctor, I am sent home without any answers. There are no medical interventions to be done, no tests that can put my mind at ease. I have to be patient. I have to allow nature to take its course, whatever that entails. I leave the emergency department with an appointment to return in three days, feeling deflated that nothing can be done except to wait.

Those three days creep by while I follow my self-prescribed bedrest. I panic at every trickle of blood. I will myself to remain calm, trying to believe that my baby might still be okay. All of my false hopes are shattered when I return to the hospital. There, a doctor, reminding me of my immigrant father, dark-skinned with a black mustache and the hint of an accent you can't quite place, stands uncomfortably by the door to my hospital bed and says, "I'm sorry, but you've lost the baby."

My sobs sound foreign and primitive, even to me. The thin, pale blue curtains provide me with little privacy, and I feel as though my pain is on display to the other patients nearby. His words reverberate around the room, echoing like a scream. With these few words, he's spoken aloud for the first time a prophecy that will define my life in the years to come.

I cling to Joey while the doctor interrupts my moment of grief.

"The good news is, you can get pregnant!" he says, much too brightly. "Miscarriages happen all the time. You're young, you can try again soon." And with that, the first dismissal of my grief for a baby who would never be born, he leaves. A nurse comes in shortly after, describing what to do if I bleed too much and where to place my hospital-issued gown before leaving. I'm given a useless pamphlet about the physical symptoms to expect during a miscarriage, and no instructions on how to live with a baby that will not.

I cry the entire way home.

Over the next few days, I take handfuls of over-the-counter painkillers and cringe whenever I have to go to the bathroom. I am unable to look away from what fills the bowl beneath me. Blood, tissue, things that remain indescribable, are all flushed away. I sob my way back to bed, certain I have flushed our baby down the toilet.

I HAVE BARELY SLEPT BY THE TIME MY NEXT APPOINTMENT arrives three days later. The grief has consumed my whole self, my body wracked with alarmingly painful physical side effects, a constant reminder of what's been lost. I return to the hospital, red-eyed and barren, waiting for a new physician to look for any remaining *products of conception* that may be lingering inside me. This is a term I will hear repeated over the weeks and years to come. One that will one day make me snap at an ultrasound technician, "That was my baby."

I undergo a painful internal ultrasound and it is in this darkened room where I am told I had been pregnant with twins.

"Twins," I breathe.

After my scan is over, I am handed a pad to put between my legs and I waddle back to my bed, wincing in pain. I pull my knees to my chest and I am sitting, stone-faced, when the doctor walks into my room. She sits on the side of my bed and I hope she is about to tell me this has all been a mistake. That these babies will be born after all and I can go home to my Pinterest nursery boards and my tiny onesie, having averted a horrible tragedy.

"I want to discuss a few things with you, Joanne," she starts. "You were told you had been pregnant with twins, correct?"

"Yes," I manage to say.

"Well, we are concerned that one baby may have implanted itself in or around your fallopian tube."

She explains how one twin had misfired, landing itself in a precarious position. Instead of taking up residency in the softness of my uterus, it had made itself at home in my fallopian tube. A rare heterotopic pregnancy, the odds of which are less than one in thirty thousand, where one twin does not cooperate and goes astray. The wild twin, our spirited child, the one who would have kept us up late with worry as a teenager.

"When this happens, we need to ensure your health is not in jeopardy," she continues. I look up in response to her carefully chosen words, and the fog of my grief lifts slightly. I look over my doctor's shoulder—she is still sitting on the edge of my bed—and I notice a sea of health-care personnel congregating outside my small room. A silent signal I have come to know, as a nurse, that a patient is in need of urgent care. "I am sending you to another hospital for an emergency surgery. Your fallopian tube could rupture, causing an internal hemorrhage, which can be life-threatening. We are sending you by ambulance right now."

I feel bewildered and I glance over at Joey, who is pale and wide-eyed, looking just as I feel. The doctor stands, nodding to the people outside my room. Two paramedics and a nurse walk past her and begin the busy work of preparing a patient for transport. Someone puts an IV into my arm and I am asked to shimmy onto a stretcher. A bag of solution fills my veins with a clear, cold fluid and the coldness creeps up my arm. I hear the *beep-beep-beep* of my heartbeat when a portable monitor is turned on. Within minutes, I am swiftly loaded into the ambulance that has been silently waiting for me.

During the drive, all I can think is, *I was going to have twins.* Tears threaten to fall, but I blink them away because I am trying to be brave. My two babies, who were the size of blueberries, are gone.

I am still trying to process the loss of not one but two children when the ambulance delivers me to the IWK hospital where I work as a pediatric nurse. I keep my head down while the paramedics wheel me through the hallways I know intimately, praying I won't run into anyone I know. I am filled with intense shame for being on the stretcher instead of beside it. A newfound vulnerability born from being a patient in a world I know only as a nurse.

It is briefly explained that I will undergo a laparoscopic procedure. The surgeon will make three small puncture wounds in my abdomen and send a camera in to find the unwieldy twin. They will use tiny instruments to remove the embryo and fix anything that has been damaged inside me as a result of my problematic pregnancy. I will also undergo a dilation and curettage (a "D and C"), a procedure to remove the last pieces of my children. When I google the surgery at home later, while recovering in bed, I cringe when I read the words used to describe the removal of my embryos. A doctor *dilates the cervix, using an absorbent rod,* which I picture being hammered in like a nail. *A curette is then inserted into the uterine cavity to scrape out the insides of the uterus.* A curette is described as *a spoon-like utensil* and when reading its description, I picture the hollowing out of a pumpkin at Halloween, its insides being slopped into a metal bowl with bare hands.

I am lying on a cold operating table staring at the metallic ceiling tiles. I try to ignore the stirrups at the bottom of the bed, the glaring reminders that once I am asleep my legs will be lifted lifelessly and strapped in. My blanket will be removed, and I will be exposed to the room. As I drift off to sleep, I place a hand over my abdomen, knowing this is the last time my babies will be inside me.

I am being tossed and turned, and I feel stretchy mesh underwear sliding up my legs. I lift my bum like a baby having its diaper changed, trying to help the detached hands snap the elastic over my hips. I open my eyes and the surgery is complete. I am no longer *with child, with children.* The pieces of my blueberry-sized babies, collected in plastic specimen containers, have been sent to the bowels of the hospital, where a pathologist will examine their remains.

I lift my shirt to look at the three fresh wounds that dot my abdomen. The only evidence I have left of their fleeting existence. I will look for those scars in the years to come when the calendar approaches my first children's would-be birthday. I will long for them to have remained angry and bright, a bold and insistent reminder that I had nearly been a mother. Yet they will fade with time, becoming barely visible to anyone except me.

The surgeon explains to me after my surgery that sometimes our bodies hold secrets deep inside. Secrets that have the ability to destroy a life, even if that life is not one's own. Something, I am told, had gone wrong shortly after *I* was conceived.

When I was a tiny cluster of cells, during the earliest of embryological stages, some of my cells fell out of line. They may have been lazy, or perhaps they received mixed messages of what they were supposed to do. Regardless, the process of turning my body from a single cell into a fully formed human was not seamless. I learn that what is happening to me as a near thirty-year-old woman was preordained the moment that first cluster of cells landed on the wall of my mother's womb.

"Your uterus is misshapen," the doctor explains. "This can lead to problems with fertility." The surgeon pulls out a pen and quickly draws two pictures on the back of a pamphlet I have been given to take home. I look back and forth between the picture of a normal uterus and the crude hand drawing of what the surgeon saw inside me. I feel like a child, trying to find the differences between two images in the back of a *Highlights* magazine, but the difference here is immediately obvious. My uterus is clearly not right.

A normal uterus, resembling the drawings I labelled as a girl in health class, is shaped like a jovial upside-down pear. Mine is like a humourless cartoon heart. There is a divot at the top, leaving a sharp point in the middle instead of the expected smooth, rounded edge. Its euphemistic term is a *heart-shaped womb*; its scientific name is a *bicornuate uterus*. I am told there is no cure for what I was born with, no pill to take, and no surgery that can fix what is wrong. This is my first miscarriage caused by my incompetent anatomy; I will endure four more.

The pamphlet describes my new diagnosis, with its original drawing on the back, and the surgeon explains how my heart-shaped womb isn't all. I have fibroids growing in my uterus, non-cancerous tumours, endometriosis, errant uterine tissue growing in odd places, and adenomyosis, the rare and poorly understood cousin to endometriosis. He tells me how each condition brings its own fertility complications and how their treatments cause more problems than solutions. Surgical scarring can make a uterus inhospitable for growing a baby, and the only definitive cure for any of these things is a total hysterectomy.

"You're lucky you got pregnant when you did," he says.

I don't feel lucky.

With a prescription in hand for drugs I never take because the post-surgical pain will be a reprieve from the whole-body pain of grief, I leave the hospital.

I am standing, squinting in the bright sunlight of a midsummer afternoon, when I wonder, *Where will my babies go when the pathologist is done with them?*

I don't dare go back inside and ask.

2

▼

I WAKE UP ON TEDDY'S FIRST BIRTHDAY FEELING EXCITED, FILLED to the brim with expectant emotion. The cold December air feels alive, as though it, too, is joyful for my son's presence. The memories of this day, one year ago, are crisp and clear. I feel as though I am reliving the day of his birth, while celebrating his birthday at the same time.

While cooking breakfast for my son, I can see myself sitting in a hospital bed in the early hours of the morning, taking pills placed neatly on a bedside tray. When cutting large, fluffy pancakes into small pieces for Teddy to shove happily into his mouth, I remember being wheeled into a darkened room where I underwent an ultrasound, my doctor looking intently for any signs of distress. When Teddy licks the sweetness of maple syrup from his fingers, cooing with delight, I can hear his heartbeat *whoosh* from the monitor the nurse strapped to my large, exposed belly. As I listened to the familiar beats of his heart that day, I craned my neck to read the bright red numbers that told me he was okay.

I no longer need numbers to tell me that my baby is alive.

Joey and I hang a string of photos on the wall that document each month since Teddy's arrival. We point to the once-mini version of the toddler he is now, showing him how much he has grown. I cannot believe a year has passed. I cannot fathom he didn't exist twelve months ago in the way he exists today. As the day progresses, I am unprepared for how momentous it all feels, how proud I am that he is turning one. I make cake and we wear party hats, singing loudly while a giant balloon, a golden

"1," floats in the background amid our still-decorated Christmas tree. We pose for photos, taking a video of him saying "Ooooh" after I blow out the candles for him.

When evening falls, Joey and I bathe Teddy together, making silly faces at him while we pour warm water over his soft skin. We pull on his pajamas, wrestling his feet into the soft striped fabric while his legs kick excitedly. I pick Teddy up and Joey kisses him goodnight. He leans over and kisses me too.

"We have a one-year-old," Joey says, his voice filled with fatherly pride. I nod, smiling back, feeling the weight of the occasion just as keenly as I feel the weight of Teddy in my arms. Joey closes the door and Teddy and I are alone to spend the last few moments of his birthday together.

We settle into the grey rocking chair that sits in the nursery; in another year we will move it to our living room, no longer needing to rock a two-year-old to sleep. I unclick the clasp on my nursing bra and Teddy latches instantly. We are attuned to each other in a way we weren't one year ago.

I look at the clock: 7:25 P.M. I watch as the seconds tick down to the moment he was pulled from my heart-shaped womb.

7:26 P.M.: I sing quietly. A watery version of "Happy Birthday."

7:27 P.M.: I audibly sob. Teddy looks up at me in the darkened room.

"It's officially your birthday, love," I whisper through tears, stroking his soft head. I close my eyes and I can feel the tugging on my body as the doctor pulled Teddy from me. The moment his screams filled the operating room with a life that didn't exist a moment before. I can hear the emotion in Joey's voice as he announced, "We have a boy!"

I rock Teddy for longer than normal that night, letting him linger on my breast, watching him drift to sleep. In all the years of trying to have a child, I didn't realize what a treasured day our son's birthday would become. This day is more important than the day I discovered I was pregnant, crying tears of hope and fear for the life that was now within me. It is bigger than the day we discovered Teddy was still alive despite the blood that came. When we saw his heartbeat flicker and his tiny limbs wave instead of a still image and the words *I'm sorry* being spoken aloud.

The day Teddy arrived safely to earth, crying with the intensity of being alive, brings tears of gratitude to my eyes. It makes me want to drop to my knees and kiss the earth for allowing me the gift of bearing this child. It balances the grief I hold for the babies I lost with the joy of mothering my son. It is when I feel the intensity of love for the child in my arms as if I am holding him for the first time all over again. When the nurse placed my three-pound baby onto my chest and I became speechless, overcome with emotion that he had somehow survived. That he is here.

I place Teddy into his crib, stroking his head, and I whisper, "I'm so glad you're here."

Before leaving, I grab his baby book from the shelf in his room. Tucking it under my arm, I close the door softly and retreat to my bed, where I write about the day, blending my detailed account of what we did with the emotions retained from the year before.

You smelled like heaven, I write, unable to separate the two days from each other. *If I were to have been given one hundred babies to choose from, I would choose you, every single time.* I cannot unwind the love I have for my toddler with the love I had for my newborn son. They are the same, knitted together tightly, strengthening with time. I am unable to separate the boy I kissed goodnight from the baby I once carried inside. He is both. The baby I longed for, the child I have.

I am so glad you are here.

3

▼

I WALK TO MY THERAPIST'S OFFICE FOR THE FIRST TIME IN THE middle of winter. I can see my breath as I walk the short distance from my car to the tall grey building that blends in with the drab winter landscape around it. The fog that hangs thick in the air is the same hue as the concrete and the once white snowbanks are now dirty from street debris. I stop for a coffee on the main floor and when the barista asks me if I want whipped cream I reply, "Sure, why not?" as if I would normally say no—except I always get the whipped cream. I want to be seen as the type of woman who usually asks for a non-fat, sugar-free, skinny latte. I care too much about what other people think of me. After he hands me my coffee, I take my time putting on the small plastic lid that never fits quite right and I envision how it might end up in the ocean someday. I make a mental note to bring my travel mug to my next appointment, if I ever have another appointment.

I hit the "up" button on the elevator in the lobby and I automatically push the number four. When I get off, I realize I have accidentally gone to my doctor's office, which happens to be in the same building. I curse the lack of stairs.

"What would everyone do in a fire?" I muse aloud in the empty hallway, looking at all the closed doors that hold a myriad of health-care facilities behind them.

The elevator dings its presence and after a quick ride two floors down, I am facing a door that leads somewhere I don't want to go. I check my watch and force myself to go inside. I walk into an inviting waiting room with soft lighting and quiet music. A kind receptionist smiles and asks if I would like a drink. I hold up my coffee cup in response and she hands me a clipboard full of paperwork to fill out while I wait.

I take a seat in the waiting room, relieved by its emptiness. As I fumble with my winter coat, I look at the papers in front of me. On the first page is a series of boxes I'm meant to fill in to indicate why I am here. I take my time ticking the three that apply and awkwardly hand the clipboard back to the receptionist, dropping the pen on the floor in the process.

I fiddle with the cardboard on my coffee cup, peeling back the edges like I do the labels on my beer bottles, and I look around the room. An iron bicycle statue sits in one corner and a quaint coffee station in another. I cross my legs and my knee bounces. I am about to reach for my phone to scroll through social media when a woman opens the door beside the main desk. She looks at the clipboard with my paperwork.

"Joanne?" she asks, looking directly at me. There is nobody else here, so I don't hesitate to nod, a tight, closed-lipped smile pasted on my face.

I stand, draping my coat over my arm, and walk toward her. She's tall, and I feel childlike beside her. She smiles quietly at me, not too broadly, which is nice, because she knows why I am here. She walks me through a short hallway, making comments about the weather, standard small talk those of us on the East Coast can't seem to resist.

The room I am ushered into is filled with beachy accoutrements that are perhaps intended to make you feel like you are at your best friend's cottage, and not inside a counselling office. There is a low, comfortable couch on one side of the room, and separating it from a pair of armchairs is a distressed coffee table. The magazines spread out in front of me have titles like *Hope* and *Finding Your Path*. I am tempted to browse through them to see if they are parodies but I don't have time to look closer. Seconds after I am settled, wondering if I put my coat in the right spot, my therapist comes into the room and sits directly across from me. She introduces herself as Heather and doesn't ask me how I am doing. We are off to a great start.

"So, you put on your form that you're here for"—she pauses briefly and looks at the papers in front of her—"Miscarriage Support, Anxiety, and Emotional Support. Can you tell me a little bit about that?" She looks up and waits for me to explain.

"Well, I just had my fourth miscarriage," I start. "Actually, I am still having it." My cheeks flush, and I cross and uncross my legs, feeling the crinkle of my diaper-sized pad as it shifts beneath me. I feel exposed and emotionally raw, like when you get a bad sunburn and even a warm breeze is painful. I want to cover my sensitive skin up in layers. I feel as though I am sitting here naked, vulnerable.

Her silence makes me uncomfortable and I ramble to fill the void. "But I have a son. He recently turned two, so I'm really quite lucky." I take a sip of my coffee, willing her to say something in return. I peel back the cardboard on my cup even further, the adhesive snaps. I slide it off, leaving my cup looking as naked as I feel.

Her head cocks to one side and she writes something on the page in front of her. I covertly try to read it.

"Could you rate the level of emotional distress you are feeling right now? On a scale of one to ten. Ten being the most distressed you have ever felt."

Without hesitating I say, "Eight."

"That's quite high," she answers, with another scratch of her pen.

I nod and purse my lips in response.

"I want you to tell me a little bit more about what's going on…If you can," she adds.

I look at my hands and feel another wave of heat wash over me. I am crying before I even speak. "Well," I say quietly. "Four feels like a lot."

"Yes. That is a lot," she replies. Her response and kind expression prompt me to continue.

"I guess I feel like I should be better at this by now. I mean, you would think after this many I'd have figured out a way to get through this."

She shakes her head. "Grief doesn't work that way. Each time we go through something traumatic, there can be a cumulative effect that can cause more pain."

I freeze after she says the word *grief.* I ruminate on it for a moment. Grief is intended for the loss of people you knew, not the physical manifestations I am dealing with. My losses feel so inconsequential compared to those who have lost someone who really existed. Their tears are meant for someone. Mine are meant for positive pregnancy tests turned negative, and bloody underwear balled on the floor. It is silly of me to even be here. So, what *am* I doing here? I feel like I am posing as a grieving mother: how can I be grieving for babies who were never born?

When in the throes of a miscarriage, I make jokes and smile through my tears, trying to portray the ever-positive image I have curated of myself. I tell most people I am doing fine because all of my losses happened early, while my heart continues to break. I am repeating phrases that have been told to me by others. After six years, I have learned what people want to hear, but these words only comfort them, not me.

My mother tells me stories of how good-natured I was as a baby. As her third child, she felt guilty that she didn't have enough alone time with me during the day. Before she went to bed, after my older siblings were asleep, she'd come into my room and wake me from my crib, ensuring we had a few minutes alone together each day. She tells me how I smiled at her when she cuddled me in the chair and how I never fussed when she put me back to sleep. A happy baby.

I receive report cards in nearly every grade with teachers' notes like *Such a happy child* and *Never stops smiling!* My parents ruffle my hair, smiling proudly, and jokingly say, "Yes, that's great, but can you read?"

As a teenager, I complete dozens of personality quizzes online. I spend the ten minutes I am allotted daily on our family computer, connected to the internet by dial-up, trying to figure out who I am. One quiz is titled "What Song Are You?" and I answer each question quickly, waiting patiently while the internet works hard to give me my results. Finally, the screen flips to the results page and I smile when I read, "Walking on Sunshine" by Katrina and the Waves. There is a poorly written paragraph describing how naturally happy I am and an animated sun with sunglasses spins around the corner of the screen. I log off, feeling content to find my self-perception reinforced by a quiz I found on the internet, and it is all there in black-and-white Comic Sans.

FOR WEEKS AFTER EACH MISCARRIAGE, I TAKE LONG SHOWERS, sobbing to the point of dry heaving; I am literally brought to my knees by my grief. I don't feel lucky that my miscarriages happened early, and I am adept at hiding the worst of my despair from everyone around me.

Except Joey.

I fight with Joey the day before I come to see Heather. Something as innocuous as dishes left on the counter has me spitting expletives at him, slamming cupboards in an outrage.

Getting out of bed these days feels impossible, and the weight of another loss has drained me of my natural optimism. I grew up with the belief that my positive, happy-go-lucky nature was an innate part of my personality; my miscarriages challenge that. And if I'm not that person, who am I?

The day of my first appointment, I tell Joey I am going to speak to a therapist. He is encouraging and hugs me before I leave. He, too, is afraid of who I am becoming. I didn't know I was capable of such anger and sadness. It frightens me to consider that maybe this is who I have been all along. That maybe my entire life has been a lie until now. Maybe my miscarriages are peeling back the layers I had kept hidden behind a sunshiny front. Maybe this is who I truly am.

With adrenaline coursing through my veins, I fight against my instinct to flee from the serenity of Heather's office, forcing myself to sip my coffee and wait for the panic to pass.

4

▼

I GREW UP BELIEVING THAT PREGNANCY COMES EASILY. For years, I took a daily birth control pill with the understanding that an unwanted pregnancy was the worst possible thing that could happen to a girl full of dreams. I wanted to be a doctor or a veterinarian in my early twenties, or if you spoke to three-year-old Joanne, a checkout lady at the grocery store. I loved hearing the *beep-beep-beep* of the food as it passed through the red light. I would sit in the seat of the grocery cart, eating the animal crackers my mother bought to placate me, and be transfixed by the woman behind the counter.

All of my goals felt so attainable until I turned twenty-seven and tried to have a baby.

Infertility was never mentioned. Issues with conception, miscarriages, faulty uteruses: these were the plotlines of movies and television shows, where ultimately a couple undergoes IVF and, inevitably, a baby is born. No one ever told me that infertility affects one in eight couples, and I lacked the insight to consider it might affect me, too. And so, I walked around for nearly three decades assuming pregnancy would come easily to me as well. I knew what I wanted out of life and I thought I knew how to get it. I had a plan, and I was under the illusion that my life was completely within my control. Fertility felt like a given, like something owed to me for following the rules.

My try-hard attitude remains a steadfast part of my personality. I feel a sense of comfort when I can exert control over the outcome of a challenge. Big exam coming up? Study hard and get an A. Want a new job? Make connections and prepare well for the interview. I realize this is a privilege, and when faced with infertility, I would struggle to learn that some things cannot be achieved through sheer will.

I EXPECTED TO BE A MOTHER THE WAY YOU EXPECT THE EARTH to keep spinning and the sun to rise each morning. It was a certainty. I was raised in a house filled with four children, pets, and a lot of noise. My siblings and I were cared for by my mother, who stayed at home until we were all school-aged, my father returning home each evening with a briefcase in hand. My neighbourhood was mostly white, suburban, and filled with middle-class families like mine. A family meant a mom, a dad, and two or more children. I wasn't provided many examples that challenged this narrow view of family, and my own mirrored the fictional television shows I watched nightly, reinforcing my singular belief. I lacked the imagination—or maybe the courage—to dream of another life for myself outside the confines of the nuclear family.

This desire for an embarrassingly traditional existence as a woman feels like it borders on being un-feminist, but what is feminism without the ability to choose? I longed to be a *normal* woman—the same *normal* I saw in my mother, my grandmother, and my friends' mothers. I wanted to exist as a wife, as a mother, and to have children fill my home completely. To wish for anything different felt scary and intimidating, because what if I failed at whatever else I tried to become?

In my diary as a child I wrote about becoming a writer, a veterinarian, a pediatric brain surgeon, each dream loftier than the last, but I always made sure to include *mother* to ensure I knew what I was most suited for. At age seven, I had names picked out for my future children—two boys and a girl—and I dreamt of my future family sitting beside each other on a couch like Russian nesting dolls out on display. I imagined my life unfolding like a 1950s suburban dream. I never considered that my life wouldn't go as I imagined it would, that I could fail at even the most banal of existences. I didn't know what it would mean to fail at the one thing it seemed I should be capable of achieving.

I MEET THE BOY I WILL MARRY WHEN I AM EIGHTEEN. IT'S THE first day of university and a swarm of freshmen buzz throughout campus with the energy that comes from being young and nearly free. We all wear the matching yellow T-shirts that have been given to us; it is a brand of sorts, allowing new students to find each other easily, though our wide eyes and fresh haircuts are proof enough. On the front of the T-shirt is written *Class of 2008*, and the back is littered with advertisements for the few restaurants and stores that our quaint university town contains.

My parents drive me the two hours to my new home at Mount Allison University: a tiny dorm room I share with a girl I have only spoken to once on the phone. It is a year before Facebook will erupt across campus and all I have to go by is a voice and a name. Our room is so small we can stand side by side with our arms stretched out and touch both walls. Our smaller-than-single beds have mattresses well-worn from other students' use and I am too young to worry about the visible stains. My parents help me unpack and I talk excitedly with my new roommate and anyone I meet in the halls; it feels like everyone is a new friend just waiting to be made.

That evening, the new students proceed across the quad to participate in a traditional commencement ceremony. We wear black gowns and instantly forget the names of all the adminis-trators on stage wearing funny hats. This ceremony is a long-standing tradition intended to mirror our graduation that will occur four years later. The chancellor of the university stands at the podium speaking about the merits of a liberal arts degree and welcomes us to his campus. He tells us to look around, to imagine ourselves four years older when we will walk across the stage having become accomplished scholars. I look around the auditorium adorned with red velvet seats and life-size paintings of regal-looking faculty members, and feel a surge of excitement for the years to come.

After the ceremony, I meet my mom on the steps of a build-ing straight out of *Harry Potter*. It has pillars and cobblestones, reminding me how far I am from my suburban home. She lingers for a moment without saying anything. A hint of sadness flashes across her face, but she smiles when she leans in to give me a hug and tells me how much she loves me. Looking back on this moment, I can imagine the many emotions she must have been feeling and how bittersweet that night must have been for her. I wish I could go back to those university steps and give my mom some words of appreciation for how much she had given me. To take a moment to acknowledge that this final push, leaving me in a new town to navigate the world alone, must have been so hard for her. I wish I had told her how grateful I was. Instead, after hugging her tightly, I simply walked away without looking back.

Every new student is placed in a group of eight other freshmen. A seemingly mature sophomore student with a clipboard and a fancy white golf shirt takes our names. We have taken off our black gowns and are once again wearing our yellow T-shirts. It is a blind group date with people we will likely never spend time with again, intended to provide us with a sense of connection while we experience the rituals of frosh week: obstacle courses, lectures, motivational speeches, and most importantly, the parties. It is the era of hazing and initiation, rituals that have since disappeared (and for good reason), but I show up to every event eager to participate. I embrace my new life full on.

I meet my group under a giant tree across from the university's quad. The new students, and our white-collared leader, are standing around awkwardly, making excited chit-chat as if they are kids at a summer camp. I join the group and answer "Halifax" when asked where I am from, even though I would have been chastised by my friends back home since I am from a suburb thirty minutes away. But this is my chance to be someone new. And tonight, I am a girl from a city. Most of the other students are from a nearby town, some from more exotic places like Toronto or Montreal. Standing in the group is a boy who smiles widely when I approach. His face radiates warmth and familiarity, and I am instantly attracted to him.

"I'm Joey," he says, extending his hand for a formal introduction.

His hand is warm when he takes mine in his, and I feel a tingle of electricity pass between us.

"Joanne," I reply, smiling back at a face I already love.

A couple of months later, we become known as "Jo and Joe," and we love the kinship of our names. When someone calls out "Joe!" we laugh when we both turn around, feeling as though our names are drawing us closer together. Our first date is spent at a coffee shop and we discuss the names we like most for our future children. Joey says he'd like to have two—a boy and a girl—and my heart is still set on three. After we marry, we marvel at how certain we had been of our future as parents, how we always knew what we wanted.

As the weeks pass, we sneak glances at each other during chemistry labs and have romantic dates sitting outside the music conservatory. We listen to students practice while they unknowingly provide the soundtrack to our evening. We spend nights entangled together on our tiny, dorm-issued beds, learning how our bodies respond to each other's touch, and we jump under the covers when one of us forgets to lock the door and a roommate walks in.

As summer vacation approaches and our final exams are completed, I am afraid our relationship is about to end. Joey's hometown is nearly three hours away from mine, and I assume he won't want to date long-distance. I figure I will be single, back in my old room, surrounded by physical reminders of the child I once was. I lack the maturity to ask him outright how he feels, or to tell him what I want, but I purchase a bus ticket for the following week that will take me to him, just in case. I want him to invite me on his own, so I don't say anything about our pending separation.

After helping me pack my parents' car, Joey leans into the passenger window to kiss me.

"So, when are you coming to visit?"

His smile makes every doubt I had disappear. The following week, I board the bus as scheduled, with a mixtape he made to keep me company.

OUR FIRST SUMMER TOGETHER IS MAGICAL. WE COMMUTE every couple of weeks and write long emails to each other twice a day. I wake in the morning and rush to my computer, anxious to read the love letter I know is waiting for me. We drive each other around our hometowns, pointing out personal monuments to each other as though offering a guided tour of our past lives. I drive him to the lake where I camped in high school, telling him how much fun I had jumping off the cliff with my friends and drinking the too-sweet vodka coolers our older siblings had bought for us. I meet his parents and brother, falling in love with the openness of his family and how they can discuss absolutely anything at the dinner table. I learn that the way to their hearts is always eating second helpings and making everyone erupt in laughter from a well-timed joke.

We make love for the first time in Joey's childhood bedroom, a room still littered with remnants of his adolescence: posters of snowboarders taped to the wall, broken toys he hasn't played with in years stashed in a corner, and a collection of bobby pins left over from a high school girlfriend. We finally speak the words out loud for how we both feel, and it seems impossible that I existed for eighteen years before meeting him.

A week after that night in Joey's bedroom, I make an appointment with my doctor to prevent an unwanted pregnancy. I drive to my doctor's office in the rusty Toyota hatchback that has been sitting idly in my parents' driveway since I left for university, the car my sister and I drove during high school that broke down constantly. The windshield wipers snapped off in the middle of a rainstorm one day, and my sister and I tried tying a hair elastic around its broken metal without success. We drove home nearly blind on the shoulder of the road, using our four-way flashers to allow cars to pass. When driving home from dance practice one afternoon, the car suddenly filled with smoke and I pulled off to the side of the road, popping the hood like my dad had shown me. When it was cool enough to open, I saw a large rubber belt sitting atop the engine. My dad drove out to meet me and we drove it inch by inch, allowing it to cool every few minutes, to a (luckily) nearby garage. I loved that car despite its tendency to render me and my sister helpless on the side of the road. When it finally became un-drivable one day, my sister framed the license plate and gave it to me as a present. I still have it—a reminder of how free I felt in my youth.

That afternoon, I tell my parents I am going to meet a friend for coffee. I have no intention of discussing my sex life with either of them—our conversations tend to steer clear of anything deeply personal—and I feel like a real adult when I fill the prescription on my own, leaving my youth behind like I would one day leave behind my first car.

Joey is even more fearful of a pregnancy than I am. Even with the promise of the birth control pill that summer, Joey insists for years that we use condoms as well. Years later, I am reminded of their aseptic scent while undergoing transvaginal ultrasounds. The ones where a tech slides a condom over the top of a comically large, dildo-shape probe and says, "Just try and relax."

Joey and I stay together throughout our entire undergrad degree, a feat that feels impossible based on the rate at which our friends meet, fall in love, and break up with each other in the same four-year period. When graduation rolls around, it is the spring of 2008. We hold hands and grin for the camera as we flip our tassels, our black robes billowing around our legs in the warm wind. Joey decides he will pursue a master's degree in Alberta. He is leaving for Edmonton three weeks after graduation. With nothing but a biology degree and the certainty that we are meant to be together, I decide to go with him.

5

▼

IT IS NIGHTTIME WHEN WE ARRIVE IN EDMONTON, ALREADY the next day back home, and we are astonished at how light the June sky remains in the prairies after dusk. Even the air feels foreign the moment we step off the plane. Fresh Alberta air is dry and crisp. My voice takes on a deep, husky tone that rattles when I speak, as though I am a heavy smoker, and the sensitive skin on my hands cracks until it bleeds. Only my trips home to the coastal air of my upbringing soften my voice and clear my skin.

We meet our new roommates, Laura and Shawn, when we arrive in the lobby of their apartment. They have rented out their extra bedroom to us, two strangers from the other side of the country, after only exchanging brief emails. We are the same age, all of us having recently graduated from university. Laura is beautiful, tall and blonde, dressed in Lululemon pants and a green hoodie. Shawn is shorter, but funny, and makes us laugh immediately with a witty comment about how little we packed. They are a friendly couple who met in university, like us.

We make small talk while we ride the claustrophobically small elevator to the fourth floor, and once inside the two-bedroom apartment, Joey and I put our two suitcases in the fully furnished room that will never feel like home. (Laura and Shawn get married just months after we meet. We see photos of their wedding posted online, their smiles genuine and hopeful. Years later, when we discover they divorced after eighteen months of marriage, Joey and I discuss if we noticed any signs of their impending separation during the time the four of us lived together. We have little experience with divorce, both his parents and mine are still happily married, and we wondered what could have led to such a quick demise of a seemingly happy relationship.)

The next day, Joey and I are wandering around our new city and we sit down at a quaint café to have breakfast. French music is playing and the servers are all wearing white and black. The oil boom is still going strong and we watch as people walk by with an ease that looks as luxurious as their handbags. While sipping our coffees, I notice a sign posted on the door that reads, *Employees Wanted. Experience Preferred.*

I had been a hostess as a teenager at a popular breakfast joint back home, wearing a starched black uniform while I expertly laughed off the sexual innuendos from coworkers twice my age. On my last day of work before leaving for university, a beloved customer of mine, Al, handed me an envelope with my name on it.

"This is for you, and only you," he said.

Al was a successful developer in town with high expectations, even for the teenager who served him at his favourite breakfast spot. He came in every day at the same time and I felt like he was always angry with me. When I began to meet his expectations—same booth facing the window, coffee poured before he sat down, breakfast special with over-easy eggs and whole wheat toast—he warmed to me. He started asking me about my life, and while he was still intimidating, our interactions were friendly.

Al smiled when he handed me the envelope. He draped his trench coat over his arm before walking out the door, the bell ringing loudly as it closed behind him. I stepped behind the counter and peered into the envelope. Three neatly placed hundred-dollar bills were tucked inside with a sticky note that read, *Good luck, Joanne.* I gasped, a three-hundred-dollar tip was unheard of, and I felt a twinge of guilt as I slid the envelope into my pocket without telling my manager. I knew he would have demanded his cut and I was honouring my customer's wishes by keeping it all, or so I told myself.

After Joey and I eat our breakfast at the little Edmonton café, I go back to our room and update my resumé, ensuring my restaurant experience is well highlighted. My recently obtained biology degree is added in like a footnote. The next day, I am hired. I call home, excited to tell my parents I have a job, since they had been wary of my moving more than halfway across the country where the prospects include nothing more than a boyfriend. They congratulate me and I appreciate that they don't ask what I am planning to do with the expensive degree I left behind in their living room.

I work at the café for two months, learning how to make lattes with fancy little designs on top and how to manage the rush of a Sunday morning brunch. I go out drinking on the weekends with Joey and our roommates, showing up for work at six in the morning with mascara under my eyes and the stench of stale beer on my breath. I know the restaurant life is not for me. Even the late nights partying lose their appeal once the summer begins to fade, and I want a job that feels meaningful.

I've always connected well with children, having dedicated my summers during university to working at a children's camp where the girls under my care would jump into the lake after me like a row of ducklings. I was the neighbourhood babysitter as a kid, feeling like a one-woman Babysitter's Club since my phone constantly rang with parents looking for a Saturday night out. I loved being adored by little humans. I cared so much about their well-being, and I got so much more out of our interactions than I am sure they ever did. I could match their energy with impromptu dance parties and always used silly voices when reading bedtime stories. I felt like I could truly be myself in the presence of a child.

I fill out a personal page on a website that links families with prospective child-care providers, giving myself a new identity as a nanny.

A few weeks later, I take the bus to a house on the West side of town where I fall in love with an eight-month-old baby who excitedly pats my leg like a drum and a two-year-old with heavy bangs who twirls around her living room, eager to show off for a stranger. I agree to join their family on the spot. I spend the next three days googling what activities I should do with a baby and what two-year-olds like to eat. I want to excel at being their nanny.

After our first week together, the three of us create our own mini family. We spend more of our waking hours together as a little trio than not. Most afternoons, we walk to the park near their house, the two-year-old dressing like Buzz Lightyear with the baby cooing happily in her stroller. I pretend they are my own, feeling proud to belong to them.

As happy as I am, I soon discover I do not enjoy the monotony of cleaning other people's clothes and floors, even if the perk is unconditional love from two little girls I adore. I need to be challenged. I am longing for something more. During my biology degree, many of my classmates wanted to become doctors. I spoke eagerly with my peers about applying to medical school, but the application deadline came and went, my paperwork incomplete on the corner of my desk. *I'll apply next year,* I told myself. I never did.

After being removed from the achievement pressure cooker of my undergraduate degree, I realize I no longer want to become a physician, that the dream to become a doctor was never truly my own. Instead, I want to connect deeply with people, children specifically, in a way that might mirror the connection I have as a nanny. I discover that with my biology degree, I can become a nurse in less than two years, and I apply to the University of Alberta after attending an information session. I take notes diligently all through their PowerPoint presentation and by the time I step onto the city bus to head home, I am certain I want to be a nurse.

After applying to nursing school, I dream about becoming a pediatric nurse. Every morning on the commute to my job as a nanny, I crane my neck to look at the children's hospital as we drive by. I imagine myself walking through the automatic doors to care for the many sick children tucked inside.

IT IS TWO YEARS LATER, DURING MY FIRST MONTH AS A PEDI-atric nurse, that I attend a lecture delivered by a prominent pediatric heart surgeon. He has flown in from California to share his experiences, having performed some of the earliest heart transplants on children. He speaks about the history of heart transplantation. How, in earlier years, monkey hearts were transplanted into humans. Our two species are alike, but not alike enough to fool our bodies into mistaking a simian heart for human. These failed transplants taught physicians how the human body has a tendency to reject anything not marked with its own DNA and how the delicate dance of preventing this rejection is as important as the surgery itself.

The surgeon tells us about his first heart transplant patient: an infant girl. He performed the risky operation as a young surgeon and only because she would have died without it. He shows us graphs and charts highlighting her rejection levels, which remained impressively low over the years. He proudly tells us that she not only survived the procedure but is now in her thirties. The surgeon pauses at this part of his lecture, taking a seat on the edge of the table in front of the room. He takes off his glasses, and begins to explain to us how much ownership he felt over his patient's heart, and by consequence, her life.

As a young surgeon, he forbade her from doing anything that might jeopardize his precious transplant. One thing, he says, that he told her she must never do, was to get pregnant. He tells the crowded auditorium how he believed a pregnancy would risk everything. His patient would have to take less of her medication, increasing the risk of organ rejection, and the extra blood volume in her body would strain her fragile organ. He says, with a subtle bow of his head, that he had never seen her as a person. When he looked at her, he could only see the four chambers of the beating heart that he felt were his.

When the woman, and the surgeon's heart, walked into his office when she was twenty-five, he was not prepared for what she was about to tell him. "I'm pregnant," she announced, defiance in her tone.

The surgeon explains how upset he was, and how he exploded with rage in his office that day. He tells us, in a voice filled with shame, how he yelled at her for jeopardizing his transplant and how foolish he felt she had been. That he refused to see the woman wrapped around his precious heart and how he didn't try to understand why she defied his orders so irrationally. He explained to her, then, how all of his orders were intended to keep her alive—how could she not care about that? The surgeon says she looked him directly in the eye and explained how her entire life had been dictated by doctors' appointments and medications and lists of things she was never to do. She had always wanted to become a mother, and her life, she felt, was worth the risk. She had gotten pregnant without telling him because she knew how much he would disapprove. She told the surgeon that her life was only worth living if she could *live*.

Her surgeon, now standing in front of us, admits how ashamed he was of how he reacted. How after she spoke, he finally saw the woman he had once held as a newborn baby. He apologized to her, and after a lot of reflection, he has grown to be proud of the decision she made and for standing up to him that day. His ego had been interfering with her life, the life he had given her, and what is the point, he asks the room full of medical professionals, to give life only to stop the person from living it? He smiles when he tells us that her pregnancy went well, that she is now the mother of two healthy children, and he is a proud godfather to both.

I went to this lecture to learn how to care for children undergoing heart transplants and about the complicated science behind organ rejection, but I only write one thing in my notebook that day. What the surgeon reminds us of, before putting his glasses back on and returning to his lecture notes.

Always see the patient, not the disease.

TWO YEARS BEFORE I ATTENDED THE SURGEON'S LECTURE, I WAS accepted into nursing school and I met Kellie during orientation. I didn't know it yet, but she would be the first of my friends to lose a baby. And she was the friend I called after my first miscarriage. When I came home from the hospital that sunny afternoon after surgery, when my blueberry-sized embryos were sent to the basement of the hospital, I dialled her number. After three rings, she answered, and I tried to speak without crying, but the familiarity of her voice had me in tears before I said a word.

"I had a miscarriage," I sob into the phone, unable to hide my emotion.

I hear a sharp inhale followed by a tearful reply, "Oh, Joanne." I sit on the floor of my darkened bedroom while we cry together on the phone for the pain we now share.

On the first day of nursing school, Kellie and I sit beside each other in our Physical Assessment course. This is the class where we will learn how to assess the human body. Our fragile-looking instructor walks into the room sporting a blonde bob and an oversized coat and announces that we are starting with breast exams. We all look around skeptically and some people laugh nervously, thinking she must be joking. We expected to start with an assessment of the head or the back, parts of the body that are much less intimate, but she is serious. We are instructed to choose a partner, so Kellie and I cling to each other, and we retreat behind curtains that are set up in the classroom to mimic a hospital room.

"I guess I'll go first," I say to Kellie, laughing uncomfortably. I take off my shirt and we listen to our teacher calling out instructions from the other side of our makeshift hospital room.

"Inspect the entire breast," she calls out, but I can barely hear above the blood pumping in my ears as a result of being so exposed. "Look for any bumps or puckering of the skin," she continues. Kellie takes a break from examining my breasts, pausing to look me in the eye, and she gives me a reassuring smile. "Now, touch the right breast and with your fingertips, palpate the tissue in small, circular motions. You're feeling for any lumps that roll beneath the skin."

Kellie rubs her hands together to warm them and asks, "Is it okay?" I nod, looking at the ceiling. Being felt up in the middle of class is not how I expected my nursing career to begin.

By the time our course ended, we had done all but expose our genitals to each other—something even our eccentric instructor must have felt would cross the line.

As a student, I listen to chests, tuning my ears to the subtle changes in breath sounds that can mean pneumonia is imminent or asthma is getting worse. The absence of sound is the most troubling of all. I put my fingertips into groins, feeling with my eyes closed for a bounding femoral pulse. I learn how to stand at a doorway, assessing my patient before ever putting a hand to skin. I smell the rusty stench of bleeding wounds, the putrid odour of infection, and how a delivery room fills with the scent of earth when a baby is born.

I discover how important seemingly mundane tasks are to the role of a nurse. The art of brushing a patient's teeth requires patience, but it keeps decay at bay and can help cleanse the palate after a patient vomits violently into a metal basin. I learn how to make a bed with army corners and a top sheet so smooth it looks as though I ran an iron across its surface. A well-made bed is not simply about aesthetics, although I know how even the sight of fresh sheets can bring calm to a bedridden existence. A well-made bed is the home of your patient: their couch, their favourite chair, their place to eat, to convalesce, and, sometimes, a toilet. The smooth surface of a bed is meant to protect a patient's delicate skin from angry bedsores that can appear from a single wrinkle. These wounds can take longer to heal than the illness that first put them in the bed. I've seen craters form on tailbones, tiny reddened circles appear on bony ankles, and a slight rip through the paper-thin thigh of an elderly woman. All from a displaced bedsheet. No amount of wound care can overshadow the importance of a smooth, well-made bed.

When I graduate, Joey, who is now working at an engineering firm, surprises me with a trip to Greece to celebrate and I am elated. Before the days of Pinterest and social media, I have photos of a Grecian landscape saved as my computer's desktop background and posted to my personal blog. We land in Athens, and after two days of touring the Acropolis and the ancient city, we take the ferry to Santorini. As our boat approaches the island, we perch on the top deck and watch as the beautiful seaside coast comes into view. The white and blue Grecian buildings dot the steep hillside like sheep in a pasture, and our eyes take a few minutes to adjust to all of the beauty reflected in the ocean below.

We take a bus to Oia, a town perched high in the hills of Santorini, and we stand among dozens of other tourists to watch the sunset. A man beside us pulls a ukulele from his backpack. After a few strums, he sings a Beatles song. When the song ends, Joey leans over and asks, "Can you play 'Yellow Submarine'?" The man smiles and plays the opening beats of the familiar melody. The entire crowd sings along, and the sun slips below the horizon as the last beats of "Yellow Submarine" echo across the water. The sunset is made all the more magical by this stranger's gift.

(When Teddy is two, he takes a keen interest in the Beatles. We credit a children's show that features Beatles songs as the source of his fascination. One day, he wanders into the living room, a blue ukulele held in his small arms, and he serenades us with his own rendition of "Yellow Submarine." He sways back and forth, tapping his foot in time to the music, and Joey and I feel as though we are watching the bright sky all over again. Now, when we speak about our evening standing on the hillside of Oia, the lines between past and present blur and we often forget that Teddy wasn't there beside us, singing along with his sweet voice.)

After spending a week in Santorini, with its brilliant ocean views and sparkling white-and-blue buildings, we take the ferry to Naxos. We disembark and sit down at a seaside restaurant where we eat freshly caught swordfish and grilled tomatoes stuffed with rice, flavoured with fresh mint and oregano. After dinner, we explore the town by climbing the hillside to where a castle stands, overlooking the sea below. We weave our way through the little village, passing shops and restaurants overflowing with tourists and locals alike. The street lights flick on as we get closer to the castle, and we can hear music coming from inside its walls.

We sit outside on a low cobblestone wall listening to the music and talk about how much it reminds us of our dates in university. When we were serenaded by unseen musicians as we fell deeply in love. We have a clear view of the ocean beneath us, the waves crashing providing a complimentary beat to the music around us. Joey pulls me in closely and kisses me long and deep. When we pull apart, he whispers into my ear, "I want to do this forever." He holds out a diamond ring that glistens, even in the dark.

"Will you marry me?" he asks.

I wrap my arms around his neck and the joy I feel renders me speechless. When I hold our newborn son in the delivery room years later, the same kind of pure elation will fill me completely, leaving room for nothing else, including words.

I wipe the tears from under my eyes while he smiles and asks, "So does that mean yes?"

I emphatically say, "Yes, of course!" And he slides the ring on my finger.

One year later, we stand in front of a barn on a hot August day, and we vow to love each other and make it through the hard times together. We dance with our friends and family, feeling so hopeful of our future. The naïveté of our youth allows us to envision that life will always be this good, and that our agreement to stay together through the hard times is not something that will be tested so soon after our wedding.

6

▼

THE WEEK BEFORE JOEY AND I GOT MARRIED, MY SISTER TOOK
me and my bridesmaids to have our fortunes told by a psychic
she found online. We rang the buzzer outside a brick apartment
complex and were ushered in by a faceless voice and the click
of the glass door being unlocked. We giggled nervously in the
hallway. A middle-aged woman with blonde curly hair wearing a
floral T-shirt and jeans opened the door. Inside her small apartment, she gestured to the round card table set up in the corner.
It was covered with a tablecloth that looked like a giant doily.
The room smelled like incense and kitty litter.

The shiny ring on my finger sparkled with the hope I had for
a happy future. The psychic knew I was getting married, and that
this outing was part of my bachelorette party. I doubt she would
have told me if she saw anything menacing coming my way. My
face was too eager, my eyes wide with a youthful innocence. I was
here to be told how happy my life was going to be.

As we sat at the small table, she told me how I was marrying
the right man. I smiled. This, I already knew. She saw the ocean,
which was vague enough to ring with meaning in my mind, and
that our wedding would be beautiful. She said she saw three
children in my future—two boys and a girl.

"No. Three boys," she said, correcting herself as her vision
became clearer. She told me to expect a child within the year.

I smiled the whole time, not shy about showing my happiness
at her predictions. I looked around her apartment. The galley
kitchen stood with dirty dishes in the sink and her TV sat on a
stand so low to the ground I imagined you'd have to lie on the
couch flat to watch it.

We left the apartment filled with the energy of being given happy fortunes and I was satisfied. I knew that what she told me would come true because there was no other way for my life to unfold. I was going to have the family I always wanted.

A YEAR AFTER OUR WEDDING, JOEY AND I DECIDE TO HAVE A baby, with the assumption that this is a choice we can make. It is early 2014 and nearly ten years have passed since we first met as teenagers. We have moved back to the East Coast, where we always envisioned our family would grow, and are continuing our careers in a place that has always felt like home. We are twenty-seven and life is full of possibility. I throw away my birth control pills and I am confident I will be pregnant within the month, so certain that the mere idea of a baby will deliver one.

A month comes and goes, and my period never arrives. I take test after test, but they all seem to shout at me angrily, *Not pregnant!* After three months of taking more pregnancy tests than I can afford, I finally start to bleed. I imagine that perhaps my body needed time to readjust since I have been taking the pill for the last eight years; I wonder if my body has gotten lazy.

This goes on for a year. After countless negative pregnancy tests and consistently unpredictable periods, I seek help from my doctor, hoping she can figure out what is wrong. I explain to Dr. Comeau how concerned I am that after a year of meticulously recording my cycles and plotting our lovemaking as though charting a course on a map, I am still not pregnant. I recount my irregular cycles and wonder if the pill is to blame. I sit on the black exam table in her office with my legs dangling over the edge like I am a child. The sheet of paper crinkles beneath me and when I shift, it tears easily as tissue paper. I pick the skin around my thumbnail while I wait for her to speak.

"Eighty percent of couples will get pregnant in the first year," Dr. Comeau explains blandly, writing notes in my chart. "And ninety percent in the first two years."

Instead of feeling reassured that I will likely be pregnant within a year, I feel defeated already. I am unsure how to handle any form of failure, especially one that is beyond my control. It is my first experience of being othered in the world of fertility and it tastes sour, like a carton of milk left in the sun. I don't want to be in that bottom twenty percent. I feel like I've failed an important life exam even though I thought I was well-prepared. According to societal expectations and medical teachings, I am in the golden age for child-bearing, so why wasn't this easy?

If a woman has a child too young, others will wonder, often out loud, whether or not she will be able to give the child a good life. If a woman has a child too old, statistics will be handed out by doctors like lollipops, suggesting that she waited too long, reminding her that after the age of thirty-five a woman's fertility wanes. Never mind the growing evidence against this societally accepted, seemingly scientific truth, or the lack of evidence that a well-supported young mother cannot rear a child successfully. I am of an age that should award me an A+ in life-planning; I am young, but not too young. I have bought into the social norms around fertility wholeheartedly, and yet, because I am in the golden age of conception, I am even more concerned that something may be wrong when Joey and I cannot conceive.

At my request, Dr. Comeau sends me for a barrage of hormone tests and Joey for a semen analysis. I have to time my blood tests according to my unpredictable cycle and I am certain the results will be bad. My natural optimism is beginning to slip away.

A month later, after all of our tests are completed, Joey and I find ourselves in a cramped examination room. Neither of us wants to sit on the paper-covered table, so we choose the two chairs across from one another, our knees touching. When Dr. Comeau comes in, we have to awkwardly swivel in our seats to allow her to reach her stool.

She holds a small stack of papers in her hands, and I feel in her momentary silence that she is bracing for what she is about to say. She glances at the paper on the top of the stack, her eyes moving quickly over the results, and says, "Everything looks normal." I exhale, unsure for how long I have been holding my breath.

"You're both young," she continues. "I'm sure it will happen soon." With that, she stands, indicating our appointment is over. We shuffle out of the room, mumbling goodbyes, feeling confused and bewildered about what we are meant to do next.

MONTHS PASS AS I TRACK MY CYCLE CAREFULLY, ANALYZING every cramp and twinge for signs of new life within me. Yet each month, I fall deeper into a sense of unease about my body's inner workings. Before we know it, it's early July. The bright morning light wakes me as the sun glistens off the water behind our house, filling our bedroom with a brilliant hue. I can't shake the dream I had the night before. I reach over to my nightstand, littered with the stack of books I am reading, and I put my glasses on—I'm legally blind without them, so until I wear them, the world is foggy and uncertain. I click on my phone and check the date on the calendar. My period is three days late. I look over at Joey, and I wake him gently.

"Joe," I whisper into his ear.

"Mmm," he replies, pulling his sleep mask off to squint at me.

"I dreamt I was pregnant." He half sits up, taking his mask off completely.

"And my period is three days late."

A smile erupts on his face and after hugging me quickly, he jumps out of bed. "I'm going to get a test!" He pulls on his sweatpants and before I've gotten out of bed, I hear the front door close and the car start.

Joey knows as well as I do that my dreams sometimes allow me to discover things I can't when I am awake, as though only in the quiet of sleep can the truth seep into my mind.

WHEN JOEY AND I ARE NEWLYWEDS, WE GO ON A HOLIDAY to London to visit our British friends. We are sleeping soundly on a mattress in the living room of our friend's flat, when I wake at 4 in the morning. It is one of those heart-pounding moments you often see in movies but rarely occurs in real life. I look over to where Joey is sleeping, my heart pumping fiercely. I have just dreamt that Joey has a brain tumour. I assess him for any signs of distress, count his breaths, watch the rise and fall of his chest. Finding nothing amiss, I force myself back to sleep.

The next morning, Joey is standing in the living room turning his BlackBerry back on. "Oh wow," he says as the notifications ding. "I have a lot of emails."

I look at him and smile, wishing he wouldn't think about work. It always takes Joey a while to settle into a vacation since his job is so demanding. But we are leaving for Paris in an hour, so I turn back to the bag I'm packing. That's when I hear it. A sound like an animal howling. I turn back toward Joey and he is still standing with his phone in his hand, but his eyes have rolled upwards, displaying only their eerie whites. The noise is coming from deep within his throat. I watch as his arms rise upward and flex toward his face, his phone dropping to the floor with a bang. His body goes rigid, shaking uncontrollably. His head cracks on the coffee table as he falls, and the sickening sound of his skull against wood makes me finally react. I begin screaming for help.

I run the few steps to where Joey is writhing on the floor, his body straight as a board, and as my friends rush into the room I yell, "He's having a seizure!" Someone dials 999 and I hear a voice saying, "Please come quickly, our friend is having a fit!" I instruct my friend, who is also a nurse, to start timing his seizure. I know the risk of brain damage from a seizure increases dramatically after five minutes, and I am praying his convulsions will stop in time

Two and a half minutes pass, and Joey stops shaking. With his body still, he begins breathing in a way I have seen in patients right before they die. His chest heaves slowly, and he exhales, emitting a *peh* sound, with his lips pursed together. His saliva, mixed with the blood from biting his tongue, begins to foam out of his mouth in a pink, frothy wave. I watch his lips turn blue and he looks like a corpse. Waxy and lifeless.

"He's not breathing!" I yell. My friend, the nurse, rubs her knuckles on Joey's sternum, trying to wake him, but he remains unaffected by the pain she is causing. I open his eyelids and see only the whites of his eyes looking back. "He's not breathing!" I yell again, to nobody in particular.

This time, my friend grabs me by the shoulders, "Joanne! He *is* breathing, look!" I look down at Joey's dusky skin and I don't believe her. Somebody thrusts a cordless phone into my hand and I instinctively hold it to my ear. "Joanne," says a calm voice with a soothing British accent, "tell me every time Joey takes a breath." I look down at Joey and I say "Breath" into the phone, feeling disconnected from the word coming out of my mouth. My mind is filled with panic for my husband who I am certain isn't breathing, but the calm voice on the other end of the phone has reinstated my nursing skills. Each time I see Joey's chest heave. I say "Breath," until the exercise has calmed my own breathing.

Moments later, Joey is thrashing, his wide eyes and enlarged pupils making him appear possessed, like a zombie. He tries to get up, but we keep him down, fearful of the damage he might cause if he stands. His eyes dart around the room, not connecting with anything, and I keep saying, "Joey! Joey!" but he doesn't answer. He claws at our arms, his body trying to flee, and it is when he is in this state, with three of us holding Joey down, that two paramedics storm into the room. They shoo us away, speaking calmly to Joey. One of them slides a probe over Joey's finger, hooking him up to a monitor, while the other inserts an IV into his arm. They take a drop of blood from the tip of his finger, measuring his blood sugar, and ask me a myriad of questions about his overall health. As they do this, Joey's body relaxes, and he comes to a seated position with his knees drawn up, his arms bracing himself on the floor. He looks like a child learning how to sit. His eyes soften, and he looks less frightened and more confused.

"What's your name, mate?" the paramedic asks him.

"Ah...Joey." He sounds unsure of his answer. Joey will later describe these early postictal moments as feeling like his brain has been wiped clean of meaning. He'll say that he can feel his brain rebooting like a computer, and how there is no metaphor to describe the void he experiences when he doesn't know who or even what he is. In those first moments, when he struggles to find the words for basic things, including his name, everything slowly comes into focus like a camera lens being adjusted.

"All right, that's good. Now, can you tell me who that is?" The paramedic points at me.

Joey looks at me, first with a slight frown, then after a few seconds, recognition washes over his face. "She's...mine," he replies, and I smile back at him in the same way I will someday smile at our son when he masters a new task. The times when I feel so proud of his ability to do things like take off his own socks.

"She's my girlfriend," Joey adds.

"Wife," I interject, feeling protective of my new title.

The two paramedics help Joey to the light grey couch a few feet away, his skin tone a near-perfect match for the pale fabric. Once he is able to tolerate sitting for a few minutes, Joey is guided by the paramedics out of the flat and into the back of an ambulance parked on the busy London street. It is sunny and warm, a nice departure from the rain we'd had the day before, and commuters are waiting at the corner for a bus that I imagine might take them to glamorous places around the city, Buckingham Palace or Big Ben. A few people look over at our parade out of my friend's flat, and I glance away when someone catches my eye.

Joey is helped onto the stretcher by one of the paramedics while the other closes the back doors, pointing to the perch I can sit on. I clip my seat belt around my middle and reach over to grab Joey's hand.

"Are you all right, love?" I ask, knowing what a ridiculous question that is.

"Where are we?" He still looks confused.

"We're in London."

His eyes grow wide with disbelief. "London?"

He looks around the ambulance, now heading toward the hospital, and he looks like he is about to vomit; sweat is pooling on his brow and he grasps the basin the paramedic left beside him. After a couple of minutes of nauseated silence, his colour returns and I speak again.

"Yes, love, London. Don't you remember coming here?"

He shakes his head slowly.

"We've been here for a week. Do you remember leaving for our trip? What about home? Do you remember Maddy?"

We had gotten Maddy the year before. I had convinced Joey we were just going to look at a litter of Havanese puppies, but I had secretly bought everything a puppy might need—dishes, dog food, a couple of toys, and a tiny collar—and stashed it all in our front closet. Once we met the puppies, I looked up at Joey while cradling a white and brown girl, and he knew we weren't leaving without her. Joey had never owned a pet, so this was his first experience loving a little thing with fur that nipped at his hands playfully and cried like a baby at night.

I was working a night shift a few days after we brought Maddy home, and after nights of Maddy crying mournfully in her kennel, Joey relented and brought her into bed with him. She never cried again. To this day, she still curls up in between us every night; our bedtime routine would feel incomplete without the sound of her jumping onto the foot of our bed and nestling herself between us. (When Teddy was an infant, we placed his bassinet close to our bed and Maddy would sigh loudly and dramatically each time he woke, as if she were the one most inconvenienced by his cries.)

In the back of the ambulance in London, I think to myself, if Joey were to remember anything, he has to remember her.

"No, I don't remember her."

Joey appears sorrowful and we sit in silence while I wonder if his memory will ever return. He looks down at his hands, his facial expression reminding me of the times I saw him studying when we were in university. Intense concentration lines his face as he tries to remember the details of his own life. "Born in the USA" by Bruce Springsteen comes on the radio and Joey looks up at the speaker and nods his head along to the beat.

"Ah," he says, "The Boss."

"You a big fan, mate?" the paramedic in the driver's seat asks

Joey, smiling in the rear-view mirror.

"Yup," Joey replies, continuing to bob along to the beat.

This is the first I have heard of my husband's love for Bruce Springsteen. We've been together nine years at this point, and I can't remember a single time when he listened to him. I smile, thinking how much I love this man without a memory and a newfound love of Springsteen.

"I remember Maddy," Joey says suddenly, turning to me. "She's back home, my parents are watching her."

"Yes!" I am ecstatic that he is now remembering more than just my face.

At the hospital, a tall, gangly resident reviews what we'd done the last several days, trying to find a cause for Joey's grand mal seizure. Joey's memory seems to have returned completely, and we explain that he had not taken any drugs, and no, this was not something that had ever happened before. The doctor sends blood and urine to test for any potential causes, likely testing for drugs since his raised eyebrows to our answers indicated he didn't think we were being entirely truthful. He has Joey do a series of neurological tests that looks a lot like the sobriety tests I remember from the cop shows I watched as a teenager. The ones where officers pulled over inebriated drivers and had them walk in a straight line, perform the alphabet backwards, all while a dashboard camera caught everything on film.

We wait for the remaining test results and I call my sister, tearing up when she answers the phone.

"It's going to be okay, Joan," she says, calling me by the nickname she always uses. "Call me back when you hear more."

I hang up and sit on the foot of Joey's bed. He is sleeping. His seizure required the same kind of energy it takes to run a marathon and he is exhausted even though it is still early in the day.

The doctor returns and I wake him.

"Well," the doctor says, "we can't find anything to have caused your fit. Sometimes these things just happen."

I scoff at his remark; I know grand mal seizures don't *just happen*.

"Aren't you going to do a scan?" I demand. "You're going to let us go, without checking his brain?" I am used to challenging doctors; my job as a nurse requires me to question even the sharpest of brains, and I am determined we will not leave without looking for the tumour I'd seen in my dream. I stare at the doctor defiantly, daring him to question me.

He looks down at me—he is well over six feet—and he adjusts his round glasses. "Are you a health-care professional?" His British accent makes him sound more polite than he likely is.

"Yes, I'm a nurse."

"Well, doing a scan isn't a bad idea, is it?" He leaves to arrange the scan and I exhale with relief, but I am fearful of what the scan might show. My dream still feels fresh, and I wonder if I might still be in it.

When Joey returns from his CT scan, which has taken a series of x-rays of his brain, we wait impatiently for the report. My toes tap audibly against the stretcher and Joey, who is not normally fazed by much, constantly shifts in the hospital bed.

The tall doctor eventually returns holding a sheet of paper. "Good news," he says. "Nothing on the scan." I squeeze Joey's hand and close my eyes with relief, grateful to be woken from my nightmare. We go back to our friend's flat and I make arrangements for us to fly home as soon as possible, while Joey sleeps the rest of the day.

Once home, Joey undergoes a series of tests and scans to search for the source of his seemingly unprompted fit. Two months after his seizure in London, he receives a call from his neurologist: she has reviewed all of his tests and wants to give us the results. I have spent these last two months panicked every time Joey didn't answer his phone right away. I would call him repeatedly until he answered, and when he'd finally pick up, I'd cry with relief that he wasn't lying helpless and alone, having another seizure. When he made a noise that sounded unusual, his throat-clearing or a groan when working out, I'd race into the other room with my phone ready to dial 911. I laid awake at night, listening for his breathing, terrified he would have another. I went to sleep trying not to picture his body, how it looked like a corpse in that moment, the moment when his body existed but he had been gone.

In the neurologist's office, the doctor lists all the tests and scans she has performed. She tells us all of the things that are normal, his blood tests, his MRI, his neurological assessment. She continues talking when I wonder, *Why didn't she mention his EEG?* Joey had undergone an EEG, or electroencephalogram, a test designed to detect the brain's electrical activity, the week prior. He'd had dozens of wires glued into his hair while a tech captured all of his brainwaves on a computer. Joey said he imagined it was likely a similar experience to being in a sensory-deprivation chamber, but one that was interrupted often by bright lights and loud noises. As his neurologist continues her speech about all of the normal results, I hear her say the dreaded word: *but.* I watch as her face turns from smiling to serious.

"Joey, your EEG showed a lot of irregularity. We believe what you have is called Juvenile Myoclonic Epilepsy." I grab Joey's hand and feel my heart drop, as though I am in an elevator plummeting down a skyscraper. I look at his face, and his expression shows more concern for me than for himself. He smiles at me, the smile that made me fall in love with him, and squeezes my hand tightly. He nods his head as though trying to say everything is going to be all right and my heart steadies, the elevator catching on the last floor before crashing.

The doctor tells us what to expect. Joey's condition is treatable but will require him to take medication vigilantly to prevent future seizures. We are lucky.

With treatment, Joey remains healthy and unrestricted by his condition. Despite having had more seizures since that day in London, we are able to live without the daily fear that he will drop to the floor without warning, and I slowly learn to not lunge at every sound or missed call. Although years have passed since our trip to England, I never forgot my foreshadowing dream about Joey's brain, even though it had gotten some of the details wrong.

JOEY WALKS BACK IN THE BEDROOM AFTER DRIVING TO THE drugstore that early July morning, and he hands me the pregnancy test I already know is going to be positive. It takes three minutes of standing in my bathroom for last night's dream to become reality.

In the days that follow, I find myself wishing I had someone who could prepare me for what is to come. I long for someone like the neurologist who explained in detail that day, while Joey and I squeezed each other's hands, how his brain lacks the ability to keep out an influx of neurotransmitters, that this is what causes his seizures. She spent an hour with us, drawing diagrams and showing us his abnormal EEG, telling us what the future would likely hold.

When we asked her why this had happened, why Joey had a brain that could render him helpless in an instant, she couldn't explain it other than simple bad luck.

7

▼

THE PHYSICAL SCARS FROM MY FIRST MISCARRIAGE ARE MOSTLY gone, unless you know exactly what to look for. I sometimes place my fingernail over their small crescent shapes and push into them slightly, trying to feel for any semblance of pain. The pain of losing those babies feels like it should have killed me, like a cartoon anvil landing on my head, but I stand, wobbling back into my previous form, and it appears to most like nothing had ever happened. Without my glasses, I can't see my scars either, but I can find each one easily with my fingertips as though I am reading Braille. I wonder why I feel so changed inside when on the outside I look so similar to my previous self.

It is several weeks since I lost my first pregnancy, since the afternoon I stood blinking in the bright sunlight of a hot summer day, and my body has not yet received the message that my babies are gone. At each of my follow-up appointments, my doctor is baffled by the pregnancy hormone that continues to show up on every test they perform. It's as though my body is also unable to let go. Hope lingers in my blood as it fills my body with longing for what it once held.

Each week, twice a week, I pull a numbered ticket from the playful-looking red dispenser mounted on the wall outside the blood lab. After answering the same questions each visit, I have my blood drawn and I wait expectantly all day to see if my body has gotten the message my babies are gone. That my womb is vacant.

The first day I go to get my blood drawn, I take a registration number and sit on one of the slick plastic chairs that line the walls of the waiting room. I keep my eyes lowered and only look up when my number is called. The ding of the monitor makes everyone stir and the number I hold is now flashing in bright red. I give the registration clerk my information and after a minute the clerk pauses, as if suddenly realizing why I am there. He leans across the desk separating us. With his head bowed, I can see a small patch of thinning hair that threatens to reveal the scalp underneath.

In a small whisper he asks, "Are you pregnant?" My cheeks flush with the heat I have come to recognize as shame. I did not expect his question.

"No. Well, not anymore."

He gives me a look filled with sympathy. He purses his lips and his eyes crinkle slightly. "Listen. Next time you come in here, you don't have to wait in line, okay? You get my attention and I'll get you right in. You shouldn't have to wait out there." He waves a hand in the direction of the waiting room, where several pregnant women await their routine bloodwork. Some have babies in strollers or are sitting alone. There are posters on the wall of mothers cradling newborns in their arms, and many people are sitting closely to their pregnant partners, their arms slung over the back of the armrests, already a family of three.

My eyes fill with tears and my throat constricts with the emotions always brimming near the surface. He is the first of the many medical professionals I have seen who recognizes the grief I am experiencing. Having someone realize that my miscarriage has been traumatic is a gift. True to his word, once I register each week, he ushers me to the back room where a lab technician slides a needle gently into my arm.

After eight weeks of this routine, I am sitting in the chair of the lab with both of my sleeves rolled up, a lab tech running her hands up and down my arms, feeling for a convenient spot to stick her needle. My damaged veins are much less cooperative than they had been that first day. I feel apologetic that her work is being impacted by my body's inability to let go of the hope of pregnancy.

"Hmmm." She looks at my bruised arms, my blood vessels blown apart by previous pokes. "I think your left arm will be best today."

"Sure," I reply, knowing she doesn't need a response.

"Little poke."

She drives the needle into my vein with her head lowered and her glasses sliding down her nose. I reach between my thighs with my free hand and pinch a fleshy part of my left leg. The pain inflicted by the needle driving into my arm collides with the pain I inflict on myself. I pinch hard, twisting the skin in my fingers, knowing my thigh will be just as bruised as my arm. I have been walking around for weeks trapped in a cycle of doctor's appointments and blood draws. I have never been asked how I am doing during any of these visits. Nobody has asked if I feel like I am drowning at night beneath a wave of grief or if I cried so hard that morning that my throat is raw, my voice hoarse. I feel like a specimen to be looked at, to be poked and prodded, all while my gaping wound is ignored, slowly bleeding out.

I feel betrayed by my body, not only for not being able to stay pregnant, but for not even miscarrying properly. But I can bruise the fuck out of my leg; at least nobody can take that from me.

After two months of bloodwork and doctor's appointments, my body finally relays the message I had been told two months earlier. My body has returned to its pre-pregnant state, even though I never will. I am told by Dr. Comeau that I am now free to try for a second pregnancy.

"Sometimes women's bodies respond well following a miscarriage," Dr. Comeau explains to me in her office. "It can sometimes be easier to conceive after a loss, and it's unlikely that you will miscarry again."

And so, we try.

Joey and I try to find solace for the pregnancy we lost by getting pregnant again. I tell myself that a new pregnancy will erase my grief and that my invisible wounds will heal if only I can become a mother. After we make love, I unexpectedly cry deep, heavy sobs. The intimacy of Joey's arms provide a safe space for me to feel everything. I am scared and hopeful, wishing nothing more than for a new life to take root.

Two weeks later, a smiley face appears on my pregnancy test, blinking in congratulations. The hope I had for a second pregnancy erupts in an instant.

I see Dr. Comeau the next day, pleading with her to do anything she can to help me keep this baby. She arranges an ultrasound, and the following day, Joey holds my hand tightly while a splat of jelly lands on my abdomen in a dimly lit room. I am seven weeks pregnant. My stomach is swirling with a mix of nervousness and morning sickness. The tech spreads the gel around in a circle and we look with anticipation at the monitor directly in front of us. She spends a minute orienting herself and the fuzzy image locks onto something. She zooms in. A tiny gummy-bear shape is floating in the darkness and Joey squeezes my hand. We meet each other's eyes and grin widely at seeing our baby on the screen.

"Watch closely," the tech says. We crane our necks. "You see that?" The image is focused on the gummy bear–like shape and we see a flicker of movement that is beating along to a song we can't hear. "That's your baby's heartbeat. Congratulations, Mom and Dad!"

Hope washes over me like I am stepping into a warm bath and lowering myself into its soothing water. I feel myself relax and the tension I'd held in my body disappears completely. Our baby has a heartbeat. After having spent the last several weeks scouring online infertility discussion boards late at night, I had learned that once a heartbeat is seen on ultrasound, the risk of miscarrying drops dramatically. Joey kisses me tenderly. We are to have our first baby after all. Dr. Comeau has told me how rare repeat miscarriages are, even for someone with a uterus like mine. And I believe her.

IT IS EARLY FALL, THE TREES PERFORMING THEIR STRIKING display of colour, and we plan to tell our families the news over

Thanksgiving. It is only days after our ultrasound and I am in my closet picking out an outfit to wear to dinner when I feel a vaguely familiar cramp. An innate combination of muscle memory and mother's intuition makes gooseflesh ripple down my arms. I go to the bathroom hesitantly, my hand on my stomach, and before I sit down, a trickle of blood blots my cotton underwear. I look at the blood filling the bowl, looking for signs of life in the inkblot Rorschach test that appears.

In the emergency department, Joey and I are brought to a private room instead of the curtained-off area we sat in before. The doctor flicks off the lights. She moves the probe around my abdomen and zooms in on a figure that no longer resembles a gummy bear. It looks like a bowl of Jell-O that has been dropped on the floor. She pauses, sighing loudly, and rotates her wand back and forth. I hear the machine click as she takes photos of my uterus, my ovaries, and what's left of my baby. Tiny thumbnails of photos fill the screen and I turn my head away from the monitor. I've seen enough.

The doctor turns on the lights and sits on the foot of my bed. Tears fall on my hospital gown in tiny splats that spread as they are absorbed into the pale blue fabric. I make no effort to wipe them away. I feel dizzy. I don't want to hear what she is about to say.

"I'm so sorry," she says softly, putting her hand on the knee I've protectively pulled to my chest. I know what she is about to say next because I saw the motionless image too. The flicker, our baby's life, was gone. "I can't find a heartbeat."

My head drops under the weight of her words, and I don't remember getting dressed or the long ride home. I don't remember the days that follow.

A week later, I am in my bathroom, squeezing my thighs tightly together to try and prevent another purge of blood and tissue. I am trying to prevent a miscarriage from happening, even though I know my baby is gone. An instinct to cling to the life that had been inside; a desire to retain the decomposing tissue as a morbid souvenir of my doomed pursuit of motherhood.

What is coming, however, cannot be abated by even the strongest of thighs. I cry out when the cramps become unbearable and I resist the urge to push for as long as I can. When I finally expel what I think could be my baby, I reach into the toilet, grabbing the bloody ruins, searching for any semblance of the child that will never be. I roll the pieces of tissue between my fingers, my hands becoming bloody. When I have thoroughly inspected each piece, unsure of what I am looking at, I gently toss the tissue back into the toilet bowl. It lands with a plop. With tears hitting the toilet seat I whisper, "I'm so sorry," and I flush it toward its final resting place amidst feces and urine, my septic tank its grave. I wash my bloodied hands for longer than necessary, watching as the rust-coloured water swirls down the drain, and I wipe my tear-stained face without glancing at myself in the mirror. I am hideous; what I have just done is hideous, and I can't face such ugliness. What kind of a woman am I if my own babies are not safe inside me?

It is weeks later when I find myself in a new hospital room. My body feels empty even though the bleeding hasn't stopped. A young resident snaps off his gloves and says, "We think your uterus is empty, but we need another scan to be sure."

I don't let him know what horrific words he has chosen, and he doesn't notice the tears in my eyes as I stare at the fluorescent light on the ceiling. He isn't aware that it took every ounce of my energy to get dressed this morning, to bring myself here.

When I arrived at the hospital for my appointment that morning, I answered the same questions I am asked every time:

No, this was not my first pregnancy.

No, I currently do not have any living children.

I don't flinch when I see the giant wand. I am now accustomed to this level of indignity. I slide it into my vagina unceremoniously, shifting to try and get comfortable with the latex condom rubbing against me, its sterile scent filling the room.

The doctor takes the wand from my hand and I jump when he pushes it in too far and he mutters, "Oops, sorry," without taking his eyes off the screen.

Several minutes later, a second doctor is brought into the room. The two doctors stand, staring at the monitor that is turned away from me. They move the wand around inside my body, gesturing to what they see on the screen, as though they are playing a video game in an arcade. Wordlessly, they remove the probe, and one of the doctors tells me to get dressed before he pulls the curtain closed.

A nurse guides me into a second room that feels like a shoddy newsroom. It has an air of sadness, as if the walls have absorbed the pain of the many women who have come before me. It has pale pink curtains and a Kleenex box sits on the side table. On the ceiling above the bed is a faded picture of a garden. I wonder who taped it there and what they thought it would accomplish. I imagine a well-intended ward aid or nurse standing on the stretcher one day and painstakingly taping the photo there so that it would be eye-level with anyone in my position. I imagine they felt as though their good deed would bring joy and calm to an often-distressing exam room. I wonder if they could have known how the now-faded garden makes this entire thing more depressing. I consider standing on the bed and ripping it down.

"Joanne," my doctor says as he walks into the exam room, the door closing behind him. He sits on the small stool directly across from me and he doesn't smile. "It looks like there is still quite a bit of tissue left in there. We will need to perform another D and C."

I nod my head, angry my body can't even miscarry properly, but I am relieved that the cramps and bleeding will finally be coming to an end.

I text Joey at work, *I need to go for surgery*. Normally my texts are filled with exclamation points and emojis, but I don't have the energy for anything other than a period.

I'm on my way, he writes back. I click off my phone and change into the Johnny shirt my nurse left for me when she went to call the OR. I fiddle with my hospital bracelet while I wait.

I wake in the recovery room, pulling a mask off my face, searching for Joey in my confusion. His hand reaches for mine and he kisses my forehead.

I RETURN TO WORK TWO DAYS AFTER MY SURGERY AND I DON'T tell anyone that I lost another baby. In the evenings after showering, I curl up at the foot of my bed in a state of catatonia. I am unable to get dressed until the cold dampness of my towel forces me to pull on my pajamas and slide under the covers.

Motherhood consumes my every thought, and I become desperate for a baby. I am unable to think of anything but getting pregnant again, so I pay to see a naturopathic doctor. They tell me to look through a binder while I wait for my appointment. It is filled with happy photos of all the clients they've helped conceive. I turn the pages quickly, not allowing myself to focus too closely at all of the cheerful, smiling families taunting me. I put the binder down and go to the bathroom. I discover that I am bleeding again, a result of my erratic hormones post-surgery, and I am caught without a pad. I wrap toilet paper around my hand like a boxer preparing for a fight, and after pulling it off expertly, I line my underwear with the makeshift pad. I unceremoniously wipe my blood off the floor and toilet seat. I go back to the waiting room and watch as the receptionist enters the bathroom after me and notices blood on the floor that I had somehow missed. My cheeks redden with shame while she mops up the mess of the baby I so desperately wanted.

In the naturopath's office, she shakes her head after I tell her what happened and asks, with blame in her eyes, "What did you expect by getting pregnant so soon after your first miscarriage?" I want to remain open-minded, but I never go back after she writes me a prescription for more fresh air.

Joey and I take a long walk on the road behind our house. The ocean is to our left, down a steep embankment, and we can hear the sound of the crashing waves. With my head on his shoulder, I admit out loud to the despair I am feeling. I had never known sadness could run so deep. I feel as though I am in a hole without even a glimmer of light and my entire world feels unrecognizable. The urge to flee is overwhelming. *I need to get away from here,* I think, but the *here* is myself, my body, something I can't escape.

"Let's go on a trip," I suggest. Surely a vacation would make up for the loss of another wanted baby—and satisfy my instinct to run. We book a last-minute Christmas trip to New York City, splurging on an expensive hotel that is well decorated for the holidays by the time we arrive. We post a video online of our trip shortly after we return home, which Joey sets to an upbeat song, and our friends make comments like *Looks amazing!* and *OMG, so jealous!* I don't comment back because I can see the sadness written in our body language. We had travelled to escape our grief, but our grief followed us. It was the uninvited guest, never falling far behind on our bike rides in Central Park, and tucking itself into our king-sized bed at night.

Grieving in a new environment can illuminate things you didn't notice before. On our trip, Joey and I discover that we are travelling in two different realms of our grief. My naturally optimistic self has turned pessimistic about the future of our family, and I am filled with a shame that will take years for me to recognize. Joey is determined to stay optimistic. We will have our baby, he is sure of it, we have simply been unlucky so far.

I am certain that my faulty uterus will never carry a child into this world safely, and instead of a baby, a deep hatred of my body gestates inside me.

When I was thirteen, I was an awkward, gangly girl. All arms and legs. It took years before even the tiniest of breasts sprouted from my chest and I wrote long, drawn-out rants in my diary, *Ugly, ugly, ugly* filling the margins. I drew a stick-figure representation of myself, lines emanating from each part like the biological drawings I later drew in my university classes. I labelled all the things that were wrong with my body—*pointy nose, misshapen teeth, small boobs*—and I lamented my inability to achieve the type of beauty I desired. I think about this drawing when, years later, I draw a cartoon depiction of my uterus that has an aggressive V-shaped unibrow, sharp teeth, and a speech bubble saying, *Good luck to anything that enters!*

"I'm going to ask you to do an exercise," Heather says to me one afternoon in her office. It is still the middle of winter and the snow from my boots has melted into a puddle on the floor beneath me. I'm no longer miscarrying my fourth baby, but my loss is still all-consuming. "It might take you a while to come around to it, but I want you to say out loud to yourself, '*There is nothing wrong with me.*'"

Since I am usually so eager to please, she waits expectantly for me to participate, but I can't help but raise my eyebrows and laugh at her suggestion.

"I can't do that," I say, between rueful laughs. Heather doesn't laugh though, and her face remains serious. I clear my throat. "I can't do that because I know it's not true. There *is* something wrong with me. I have the diagnoses to prove it, and also, I am sitting here on this couch, so isn't that proof enough?"

Heather sits up straighter in her chair, putting her papers face down on her lap. "I need you to do this one thing, even though you don't agree with it right now. I'm asking that you humour me. I need you to hear the truth before you can believe it. I can get you part of the way, but you're going to have to do the rest of the work on your own."

My tongue feels dry and thick, as if it will swell, fill my mouth like a gag, and suffocate me. *I can't say it*—the words won't come. Heather waits patiently as I look up at the ceiling, the window, the door, wishing to run from this room and never come back. I want to do anything but sit on this couch with Heather's eyes taking in this broken, vulnerable person I've become.

I can't say it.

I close my eyes briefly and when I open them, I look back at Heather's kind face. As my eyes fill with tears, her features go blurry, like she is being erased.

"I can't."

She leans over the coffee table and pushes the tissue box closer to me as I sob, feeling the pain of every hurtful thing I've ever thought about myself. It's as though I am being crushed, that the couch I am sitting on will open up beneath the weight of my pain, swallow me whole, and I will disappear entirely. Heather stays silent and my words seem to bounce around the room, whispering like a mantra that only I can hear. *I can't. I can't. I can't.* I am damaged, broken, unable to speak the words that I need to hear myself say. The very words that, she believes, will heal me.

Our session comes to an end with Heather asking me to write the words down in my journal. In a messy, emotion-filled scrawl, I write, *I somehow need to believe that there is nothing wrong with me. I'm not sure I will ever believe that to be true.* I close my leather-bound journal and leave her office with my shoulders rounded, my head bent down in shame.

After I get home from my session with Heather that night, I think of all the ways I blame myself for my miscarriages and how ashamed I am as a woman, as a mother. The shame that I have killed so many babies just by the simple act of being their mother. How I have been pregnant so many times, and yet I only have one child. I feel my shame stretch and grow when my doctors ask me if I *really* want to keep trying for more children. I nurture that feeling like you would a houseplant, watering it and giving it a warm place to grow. I feed my shame with every negative thing I think about my body and I see myself as a bad person, a bad mother. A woman who has caused so much pain and destruction simply by being born.

8

▼

WHEN WE RETURN HOME FROM NEW YORK CITY, I CAN'T WAIT
for the year to be over. I want to leave the pain behind. When the
calendar flips over to 2016, I am surprised to discover that I long
for the bereaved days of the past year. I miss the days when I was
swallowed by grief because it meant it hadn't all been a dream.
It had been real. With every month between me and my losses,
and nothing to show for my miscarriages, my memory becomes
blurred. By losing the details I had clung to so fervently, it feels
like I am losing my babies all over again. I want the pain back,
to remind me I didn't imagine it all.

In early 2016, I am interviewed on a local podcast called *Sickboy*
about my experiences with infertility. It is hosted by a man with
cystic fibrosis and his two friends. They help normalize talking
about things that are often considered taboo or unspeakable, like
miscarriages. The three men laugh and joke with each guest while
they navigate stories about illness and death. One afternoon in
January, I am scrolling through Facebook and I come across an
article *Sickboy* has shared about a woman who had a miscarriage.
I read it with tears in my eyes, reading parts aloud to Joey, who
nods his head in agreement when the author's words resonate
with him as well. It is the first time we have felt understood in
months. I submit a form to be included as a guest that night and,
even in the wake of the article they posted, I am surprised when
they call me the next day. They want to hear what a miscarriage
is like and to listen to my story.

I drive to a black-and-white house one night, where I put
on headphones and speak to three young guys about the most

intimate details of my life. Their open and honest questions are refreshing, and I feel comforted by their empathy. We laugh while I tell them about my experiences. About the absurdity of transvaginal ultrasounds and the way people treat you like you're infectious when you're grieving. Laughter had been missing from my life, and when I leave their house I feel lighter, unburdened by the shame of keeping my miscarriages private.

When my episode airs, many coworkers, friends, and acquaintances reach out to me, some confiding in me that they are going through similar challenges. A co-worker pulls me aside one day at the hospital and quietly tells me, "I'm the same as you. Only I can't talk about it." She smiles sadly and I give her a hug because I had no idea. We never have any idea. We keep our sadness hidden because infertility can feel shameful. We muscle through doctor's appointments and unexplained missed days at work, and we show up regularly for painful procedures because we have no other choice.

IN SPITE OF THE BRIEF RELEASE OF SHARING MY STORY ON *Sickboy*—and the unexpected side effects of outing myself as a woman who is struggling with infertility—once the New Year rolls around, my desperation to become a mother begins to take over my life. I do not want another year to pass without having a baby of my own to hold. I need to do something to bring me closer to motherhood. Adoption feels like the natural next step, since IVF is not an option for a woman with a less-than-perfect uterus. I can't do a thing about my body, but I know how to do homework. I know how to research and fill out applications and I dive head-first into my new life plan. *Our* life plan.

I become all-consumed with my new obsession. I read everything I can about adoption, poring over books about trauma-informed parenting and raising an adopted child. I fantasize about the day Joey and I receive the call telling us that we are parents. With every box ticked off my lengthy adoption to-do list, I feel closer to meeting my child, like a woman marking off the weeks of her pregnancy.

I find a social worker who interviews me and Joey, asking us intimate questions separately, and then again together. She is looking for discrepancies, searching for the cracks in our marriage. We have to prove that we are stable, that we can parent a child. I check all of the boxes that say I am meant to be a mother. I even admit to the social worker in what feels like a generous moment of truth that, yes, I smoked weed once in university—*look how honest I am being, displaying my faults!* In reality, I am covering my wounds beneath a layer of perfection, like a fresh blanket of snow covering muddy ground. I am smiling in her presence, ignoring the nagging in my stomach that's telling me this doesn't feel quite right. That maybe I am using adoption as a way to survive my grief. That I actually long to be pregnant again, and how I'm not the image of perfection I'm trying to convey. Snow eventually melts, after all, revealing the ground beneath for what it's always been. We leave our interview with the affirmation of just how much we deserve to be parents. I hold in my hands the proof of our pending parenthood: a signed paper that says I am meant to be a mother.

After our interview, I spend a hectic few months researching and calling every adoption agency in the country. Joey and I are sitting in the kitchen one evening while I conduct a meeting of sorts. I am reviewing everything I've learned and what the plan will be moving forward. I have created a series of Excel spreadsheets on which agencies we can apply to, which international countries have Hague-approved programs and will accept an adoptive father with a known medical condition and a couple who cannot prove total infertility on paper. Many countries want completely infertile couples, and fathers without epilepsy, so our list is smaller than most. After going over all of the details, I look at Joey, who appears disinterested.

"You know," I say, with more than a hint of anger in my voice, "I'd love it if you were more involved in this."

"I am involved," Joey says with a sigh. "I just don't feel the same urgency that you do."

"Well, I'm almost thirty and it could take years for me to even get to the point where I can adopt, so I have to start now."

"But we don't even know if we can't have children yet."

"I don't care!" I yell. "I already had two miscarriages, and something is *wrong* with me. I need to do something." In my desperation I don't notice how callously I have left him out of my entire argument. I am so consumed by my own grief and need that I don't realize how far we have drifted apart.

"What if we continued to try or..." Joey pauses before he continues, softer this time. "What if we didn't have children at all?"

I snap like an animal gone rabid. My former self is gone; she is sitting some place deep inside me, cowering, while the animal in me comes to life. I feel the hairs on my arms stand up, like the scruff of a cougar's neck, and I do all but display my teeth in an ugly snarl.

"I am adopting with or without you, Joey. I need to become a mother. I can't explain it any more simply than that. If you aren't willing to become a parent with me, I need to do this on my own."

IN FIRST GRADE, THE SCHOOL I ATTENDED WAS A SMALL BRICK building that didn't have room for a gymnasium, so the end of the hallway was converted into a makeshift space where the students could expend their pent-up energy during the winter months. My classroom was in a portable building that had been built to house the growing population of our neighbourhood.

During recess one day, a boy in my class, James, was standing alone in the middle of the gravel playground. James and I were not friends, but I could tell he was upset by the way he was standing so still, not moving an inch. As I walked closer, I could see tears rolling down his cheeks and his arms lax by his sides. I went over to him and gingerly put my hand on his shoulder.

"Are you okay?" I asked, careful not to get too close to the snot running out of his nose.

In between sobs, and unable to speak, James shook his head no. He swiped his face with the sleeve of his navy-blue turtleneck.

I grimaced at the slimy stain left in its wake like a slug trail. Snotty sleeve aside, I walked James to the steps of our portable classroom, searching for our teacher. I guided him inside with my hand tucked into my sleeve. Once inside the classroom, the sounds of the other kids were muffled and his sobs grew louder. I felt uncomfortable, realizing we were now alone. We sat on two child-sized red chairs and I looked around helplessly for my teacher, but she was nowhere in sight.

Finally, James took a breath in between sobs and said, "My baby brother just died."

He put his hands on his lap and picked at the dirty skin around fingernails that were red and raw from either impetigo or continued self-abuse. I had never heard of babies dying before. I patted his elbow, careful to avoid the now hardened stain on his shirt, and I didn't say a word. The end-of-recess bell went off loudly then, echoing in the near-empty classroom. The doors swung open as the other students filed in, and when my teacher appeared, she swooped in and took James out of the room.

I was left to think about this moment alone, to try and process what he'd told me. I had never seen grief in another person before, and even my six-year-old self was curious about the way in which it could bubble to the surface, paralyzing someone in its wake. Even though it was uncomfortable, I felt a strong desire to stay beside him in that classroom. James knew he needed something, but he couldn't verbalize what that something was. I knew I was supposed to do something, but I didn't know what. We were both lost in that moment, but at least we were lost together.

My first brush with grief was a glimpse, but an immensely powerful one. I walked away from school that day feeling such sadness for James and his baby brother who was no longer alive. We never spoke about that day, but I felt forever connected to him. I can feel his grief within my own heart even today, and I am grateful for the lesson he taught me. That to sit with a person in their grief is a powerful gift. No words or actions can overpower the simple act of letting someone know they are not alone.

IN THE KITCHEN, AFTER I'VE FEROCIOUSLY HANDED JOEY AN ultimatum for our future, he cries, realizing a canyon has opened up between us. He is steadfast on the side of optimism and hope; I am unable to see past my grief. I forget about the woman cowering inside me and I don't consider that perhaps there is a better way for us to do this, as a couple. That we should be making decisions together.

After our fight, Joey hugs me and never again questions my desire to adopt. His love for me never wavers, despite how I am treating him. I am like James, broken beneath the weight of grief but unable to ask for what I need. Joey provides me with the solace of not being alone, a gift above any other. We begin preparing for a life that will bring us a child through adoption. But grief is making my decisions for me, and the anger I feel toward my body is now leeching into my marriage.

MONTHS INTO OUR ADOPTION PLANNING, I TURN THIRTY. JOEY rents a cottage for the weekend to celebrate. We pack our car and drive two hours to the beachfront property. Our friends arrive shortly after and we play washer-toss, drink beer, and eat barbecued hamburgers while we listen to the roar of the ocean nearby. We walk along the beach littered with the broken lobster traps and seaweed that the ocean tossed ashore during the colder months. We wear jackets and hats, the early May wind frigid along the water. We laugh easily as friends who have known each other a long time do. We play drinking games we remember from our time in university and I tumble into the looseness of getting drunk, not allowing myself to think about what morning will bring.

As the night goes on, we get louder and we are all dancing, swaying in the small living room. We play songs from our youth, belting out lyrics we learned by reading the inserts of cassettes and CDs. I take out my phone and put on Jenny Lewis, turning up the volume while I pour myself another drink. I had fallen in love with her recent single, "Just One of the Guys," where she sings about getting older, clocks ticking, and the contemplation of motherhood. I play it on repeat whenever I am alone. Tonight,

I stand on the coffee table in our cottage, dancing, and waiting for the line that has become a mantra to my barren self: *When I look at myself all I can see, I'm just another lady without a baby.* The catchy tune is the antithesis to the way I feel about the words I am singing, a reclamation of my sadness. It is cathartic to say these words out loud, under the guise of a song, and it is the only way I can see myself since my two miscarriages.

I had never worried much about aging, not many twenty-year-olds do, but turning thirty feels like a shift. I still pluck the few grey hairs that will eventually spread and the crow's feet around my eyes are barely visible, but I can hear the ticking clock that Jenny Lewis sings about. I go to bed dizzy but happy to be surrounded with my friends, singing and dancing like we did a decade ago.

A week later, I go to a tattoo shop. Perhaps it is turning thirty that makes me book the appointment, but I feel certain I want to mark my body with something beautiful, instead of the scars that had begun to grow there months earlier. I hold out my arm while the artist imprints a black image of baby's breath on my forearm. When it's done, I pull my arm toward my body, the way you cradle a baby, and the top of the flower rests exactly where a newborn's head would. I can't hold my babies, but I can hold this tattoo as a reminder of their brief existence.

One year later, when I turn thirty-one, I will celebrate my birthday at home with Joey and our four-month-old son. We will snap a picture in front of my birthday cake, Teddy in my tattooed arm. I will still listen to the Jenny Lewis song on occasion and remember turning thirty, feeling the weight of the year before, not knowing I will be pregnant within a month with my son.

JUNE IS UNSEASONABLY WARM THAT YEAR, AND I AM SITTING cross-legged on the hardwood floor with piles of well-organized adoption paperwork. After putting together each stack, I pat each one like the top of a child's head, praising it for being complete. I sit amid the stacks of papers and I am pleased because all I have to do now is send them to our agency and then wait for our child.

I reach for the box that is labelled and waiting to ship my precious cargo, but as I stretch my arms, I notice my breasts are sore. I grab my phone off the table to check the date, leaving the box untouched, forgotten. My period is late.

Instead of mailing in our paperwork that afternoon, I drive to the drugstore. Just minutes later, I am sitting on the edge of the tub in our bathroom staring in disbelief at the pregnancy test in my shaking hands. Even with tears blurring my vision, I can clearly see the two pink lines in the white plastic window. I am pregnant for the third time.

9

▼

JOEY IS AWAY WHEN I LEARN I AM PREGNANT AGAIN. SITTING in the bathroom, I let my tears fall readily while I try to breathe through my intense fear. I feel like I am walking on a frozen lake, listening to the creaks and groans beneath me, trying to get to the other side before the ice cracks open and I tumble into the icy waters below. I want this baby so badly the second those two lines appear, it makes my heart ache.

I barely sleep in anticipation of Joey's arrival the next morning, Father's Day. I meet him at the door, and I can't contain my excitement. "I have a present for you!"

He looks puzzled but follows as I direct him to a small package sitting atop our coffee table. He sits on the couch and I sit beside him, trying not to open it for him. He opens the gift, a small book titled *Stuff Every Dad Should Know*. Joey smiles, thinking this is because our adoption paperwork had been sent in. He doesn't know that the box is still sitting on my desk in the other room.

"Thanks, Jo," he says, giving me a hug.

"No, there's more. Open the cover!" I thrust the book back into his hands.

Joey opens the book and his eyes grow wide. I had inscribed the book with, *All my fingers and toes are crossed that the third time's the charm. You're going to be a dad!* Joey looks at me for confirmation and I nod my head with my hand resting on my stomach. His eyes fill with tears and he runs his hands through his hair, a sign I have come to recognize as his own display of fear, and we weep together.

Joey and I discuss what we should do with our adoption application waiting to be sent. We know we can't adopt with a newborn, a house with an infant being far too chaotic for an adopted child, but we aren't yet sure if we will have a newborn in nine months. We decide to wait and see what happens, keeping our box ready.

During those first couple of weeks of being pregnant, Joey and I attend a previously booked adoption-training session, and I feel guilty for hiding my pregnancy from the other couples. I feel like a fraud sitting amid a group of hopeful parents, thinking that no one else is likely carrying an embryo the size of a raspberry, the unaccounted-for member in the group.

A week after our session, I am eight weeks pregnant. I am getting ready for a night shift when I feel the now familiar pains of a contraction ripple across my abdomen. I clutch my stomach nervously and tie my shoes. I am worried this is the beginning of another miscarriage, but I want to pretend that nothing is wrong, as though by ignoring it, it won't happen.

I am about to head out the door when I have to run to the bathroom. I close my eyes. When I open them, I see an ominous red watercolour staring back. I stifle a sob, resting my head in my hands. The frozen lake has cracked beneath me, and I am submerged.

From the bathroom I call my best friend, who works in the same unit, and tell her what is happening. I beg her to work for me, not wanting to leave the unit short-staffed while I navigate the early stages of my third miscarriage. I hear a sad sigh on the other end of the phone.

"Oh, Joanne, of course," she replies gently. "I'm so sorry this is happening again. Let me know how you're doing, okay?" I thank her profusely and then call work to let them know my last-minute change of plans. I ignore their questions about my well-being.

I change out of my scrubs and put on my miscarriage outfit: a loose-fitting pink striped shirt and black pants. An outfit comfortable enough for the long emergency room visit I know awaits me. Pants dark enough to conceal any bloodstains and a shirt that can easily have its sleeves rolled up for bloodwork. I pack an extra couple of pairs of underwear in my purse, and I glance at myself in the mirror. My eyes are already filled with grief and my dilated pupils reveal the adrenaline coursing through my veins. I dread what I have to do next. I look away quickly and I turn off the lights. I walk downstairs to where Joey is sitting on the couch and he looks up, confused, since I am no longer wearing my scrubs.

"Do you not have to work?"

"I'm bleeding."

His face falls as he registers what I am telling him, and he walks over to where I am standing, wrapping his arms tightly around me. My arms remain straight by my sides, limp and lifeless like overcooked noodles. I am trying to numb myself from feeling anything about this miscarriage. *If I can perform these rituals flatly,* I think, *I will come out unscathed.*

"I have to go to emerg," I say, pulling away from him abruptly, walking to the front door.

"I'm coming with you." Joey follows me and grabs his keys that jingle when he holds the door open for me. His gesture is less chivalrous and more reminiscent of how you might hold the door open for your elderly grandmother recovering from hip surgery. While walking to the car, I feel a wave of resignation wash over me, that this is to be the outcome of every pregnancy. I feel defeated and ashamed that I had been so hopeful about this new life only minutes earlier.

I sit in the passenger seat with my knees pulled to my chest and I talk about what we will do after I have my next D and C. I discuss the pros and cons of taking more time off work and how I can send in our adoption paperwork the next day. Joey interrupts me.

"Why aren't you more upset?" he demands, keeping his eyes on the road.

"I am," I reply sharply. "I am just tired of it always ending this way."

We drive the rest of the way in silence while I stare out the window, wiping away hot tears. I am so angry. Angry at my body for doing this again. Angry that I even bothered to get pregnant for the third time. Angry at Joey for his inability to comfort me, even though in this moment, nothing could. When we arrive at the hospital, I walk three steps ahead of Joey and push away his hand as it reaches for mine, refusing to soften beneath his touch.

A nurse assesses me while I explain that I am having my third miscarriage, and then sends me and Joey to the waiting room. We sit in the corner and I stare blankly ahead, stoic and unflinching with every cramp that ripples through my body. After sitting stiffly for an hour, I feel the first rush of sadness break through my anger. The shell I had encased myself within is cracking under the weight of grief, and I lean into Joey while he puts his arm around my shoulders. We stay like this for hours, only interrupted by my trips to the bathroom. It is a scene that now feels as routine to me as a dental cleaning. I return from the bathroom and resume my position, filled with a deeper sense of defeat each time. I calculate the pads I am bleeding through, trying to determine the likelihood that my baby is still alive, and I will myself to let go of any hope I have left for their survival.

After several hours of waiting, a nurse appears in the doorway.

"Excuse me, everyone," she says loudly. We all look up wearily, many of us have been waiting for hours. "We are currently at capacity," she continues in a commanding voice. "I have a letter for each of you." She lifts her arms slightly, cradling a stack of papers. "On each one of these is a set of instructions. Based on your assessment with the triage nurse, the letter will direct you as to what you should do."

One by one she calls out names and people walk over, or hobble depending on their injuries, to retrieve their personalized sheet. She hands out three different colours of standard forms: red, yellow, and green. The red sheet tells people they will be seen immediately; their illness or injury meets the definition of a true emergency. The yellow sheet says you need to stay to be seen, but you will still need to wait. The green sheet instructs you to follow up with a family physician the next day because your injury or illness does not warrant an emergency visit. I watch as a few people with green sheets in their hands leave the waiting room hastily, grabbing coats with a snap off the backs off chairs, disappearing beyond the double set of glass doors that takes them outside.

When the nurse calls my name, I am handed a yellow sheet. *How fitting*, I think miserably. Miscarriages are not an emergency, in the vast majority of cases, regardless of how they feel. Nothing can be done, after all. They are a confusing mixture of internal panic and external calm. It's as though I am being told to calm down by everyone around me, while my body sounds a blaring alarm I can't turn off. Almost immediately, after sitting back beside Joey in our still-warm chairs. I turn to him and say, "I don't want to wait any longer. Let's go." Once again, I am overcome with the urgency to run.

"But what about your shot?" Joey asks with concern on his face.

We had learned by now that due to my negative blood type, I have to receive a blood product within seventy-two hours of the first signs of a miscarriage. The shot is intended to help protect the future of subsequent pregnancies. Without the injection, which requires me to drop my pants and bend over like a prisoner in front of a nurse, my body's immune system has the potential to attack and destroy any future baby that lands in my womb. It is a cruel twist of nature that means I do not have the luxury—if you can call it that—of miscarrying at home without the need for any urgent medical care.

"I'll go see Dr. Comeau tomorrow or I'll come back to the hospital, I don't know. I have a couple of days to get it. I just can't sit here anymore." The oxygen in the waiting room seems to have dissipated, my heartbeat racing with my body's desire to flee. I stand, grab my bag, and walk away, ignoring Joey's objections.

I pop my head into the triage room as I am leaving. "Excuse me," I say. The nurse looks up, appears to be annoyed since she likely thinks I am going to ask when I will be seen. I notice a sign pasted above her head that reads, *We do not have any information on wait times. Please wait until your name is called.* "I'm going to head out." I turn away from her to head to the front door.

"Wait," she says. "You have to get your shot." I wonder if Joey told her to say that.

"I have three days. I'll figure it out." I shrug my shoulders and I walk to where Joey is standing in front of the double sliding doors. As soon as I fall in step beside him, my face crumples and I let out a sob. He puts his arm around me and guides me out into the fresh air, passing people who are curiously watching the scene unfold. I leave the waiting room with the sounds of my grief echoing off the walls. Joey helps me into the car, and I cry the entire way home.

The next day, I am being examined by Dr. Comeau. "I'm sorry, Joanne," she says. "This is another miscarriage." She flicks her bloodied gloves into the garbage can and I shift on the paper sheet trying to cover myself. "Maybe there is more going on with you than we know. It's unusual to have three miscarriages in a row, even with your uterus." I stare blankly back because I can't think of anything to say. She calls the hospital requesting an urgent ultrasound.

Joey meets me in the waiting room. He holds my hand tightly while I wait to register. I stare at my feet, trying hard to ignore the happily pregnant couples who are likely filled with excitement for their own ultrasounds. I am so jealous of all of them that I feel it physically. I feel the familiar burn of shame that I will never be one of them.

My registration number is called, and I am handed a clipboard with a questionnaire asking me to describe how far along I am and to indicate a reason for the scan. I want to scream and throw the clipboard across the room, but I calmly take the cap off my pen and begin to fill in the blanks. My knuckles turn white from gripping the pen so tightly and I write *ZERO* in all caps in the box asking me how many living children I have. I slap the clipboard loudly onto the counter, and the woman clicking on her keyboard behind it jumps. She looks at me with a furrow in her brow and I turn away without a word.

When I am called into the ultrasound room, the tech is wearing bright pink scrubs and is extraordinarily chipper. "How is everyone doing today?" she asks with a smile that indicates she has no clue why we are here.

"You can read my chart," I say flatly, assuming the position on the bed without any direction. I lay supine, lifting my shirt and rolling down the top of my pants. I stare at the blank ceiling. Her head cocks slightly to one side and she looks at the clipboard in front of her. I sense a moment of recognition, but I turn my head before I can see the pity I assume is about to flash across her face.

"Do you want me to turn off the parent monitor?" she asks sheepishly.

I am well versed in ultrasound rooms by now. In every one, there are two monitors: one for the tech to watch while they capture all the images required, and another facing the stretcher where the patient lies, where I lie now, with Joey beside me perched on a stool. The parent monitor is specifically for the expectant parents' view, so they can comment on who the grainy image of their baby looks more like and whether or not they can see a penis.

Before Joey can say anything, I answer sharply, "No. Leave it on."

She squirts the jelly onto my abdomen and performs the scan in silence. Joey and I fix our eyes to the screen in front of us. The tech focuses in on the small gummy-bear shape we know is our baby. She zooms in and holds the camera steady. A tiny flicker in the middle of the gummy bear comes into view. I nearly sit, wanting to take a closer look, but I squeeze Joey's hand instead. With my heart racing I look at Joey, and I recognize in his widened eyes that he is seeing the same thing too. *Oh my god*, I think. *Could our baby still be alive?*

With my heart pounding, I watch with wonder as the tech takes more and more photos of a wiggling little baby with its own heart beating. I feel hope wrap itself around my shoulders and it takes every ounce of willpower not to shake the tech and demand an answer. When she is done, I use my elbows to prop myself into a half-crunch position and I look at her expectantly, even though I know she isn't allowed to tell me anything.

"So?" I demand with a still-irritated tone to my voice. My fear and anxiety bubbles to the surface as anger directed her way.

"Your doctor will call you within eight hours to give you the results," she says sunnily, repeating a script she must perform many times a day. She cleans her equipment, indicating our appointment is over, when I interrupt her work.

"No," I snap. "We are here to find out if this is another miscarriage. You are going to go get a doctor now and have them tell us what's going on."

The tech looks surprised at the tone I have taken. She leaves the room mumbling that she will try and get the radiologist.

"Did you see that?" I ask Joey, sitting upright in the bed, chewing my nails aggressively. They will be short, sore nubs by the time we leave the hospital.

"I did," he says, running his hands through his hair. "What is going on?"

After a few minutes of sitting in anxious silence, a radiologist walks in with the tech following close behind. "I heard you wanted to have an answer now," the doctor says, glancing back at the tech who dared interrupt her work.

"Well, this is my third pregnancy and I can't wait eight hours," I explain.

"The baby is fine," the doctor replies. "You have what's called a subchorionic hematoma. A bruise has formed between the placenta and your uterus. That is what is causing the bleeding, but everything looks fine with the baby right now. This isn't a miscarriage yet. You will have to see your doctor for more detail than that." She leaves the room abruptly, but I hardly notice.

Our baby is fine.

I replay her words over and over in my head. I look at Joey, who is silently sobbing. He climbs onto the stretcher beside me and I feel his arms embrace me with intensity as his body shakes with emotion. I don't know when the technician left the room and I can't remember how long we stayed like that. Nothing else mattered because our baby was fine.

Our baby.

10

▼

Dr. Comeau calls after the ultrasound. My pregnancy has a fifty percent chance of survival, and if I am still pregnant after twelve weeks—the word *if* like a sucker punch—my odds will improve, but only slightly. With all of my diagnoses, history of miscarriages, and now, the bruising on my placenta, I have received a new title which will be printed below my name on every hospital chart for the months to come: *High-Risk Pregnancy.* I feel as though I am a tightrope walker who removes the safety net before their act, the audience below gasping with every shaky step I take, wondering if they are watching a beautiful act of bravery or a careless act of idiocy. Dr. Comeau prescribes hormones intended to help improve the health of my womb, but every time I go to the bathroom, I hold my breath. I put on my miscarriage outfit almost every day, assuming each day of my pregnancy will be the last.

Joey goes to Iceland when I am three months pregnant. He has long wanted to tackle a solo hike, and the year of miscarriages and turning thirty pushed him to finally book the trip. Two months before his departure, we found out I was pregnant. I insisted he still go. We didn't yet know the fate of this baby, and if, by chance, we had a baby in nine months, a solo hiking trip wouldn't be easy to do anytime soon.

He plans his route meticulously, mapping out his course and weighing each item of his gear with a scale. He calculates the perfect number of calories needed for his body mass and buys food accordingly. Our dining room is filled with hiking gear for weeks and he shows me how to follow his GPS tracker on my laptop. He packs and unpacks his bag, rolling and tucking things in new places, seeking the most efficient arrangement of gear. He can't decide if he should take a jar of peanut butter or not, contemplating the gain of extra calories against the cost of its weight on his back.

He leaves in early September. I kiss him at the door and tell him how proud I am he is about to accomplish a long-held dream of his. He cradles my belly, kissing me back, and smiles before getting into the car. The silence of our house is unsettling with him gone. I can no longer rely on him to help push my anxious thoughts away. I pace, try reading a book, turn the TV on and off. I settle on writing in my journal about how trapped I feel in my body, wishing I were Joey. Even though a gruelling hiking trip has never been something I wanted to do, I am envious of his freedom, his ability to control even the precise weight of his pack.

When Joey sends me his first message from Iceland, I log into the GPS tracker and his dot lights up on the monitor as we speak. I touch the dot, listening to Joey's voice describe the basecamp where he is staying, and I imagine I am with him. I click through the photos he sends me of the hot springs he visits, and I picture myself bundling up with him against the cold. He departs the next morning on his hike. As Joey's coordinates move across the rocky terrain, I follow along. Each night after setting up his tent, he sends me a message, updating me on his day. He is exhilarated from the effort, dealing with the harsh conditions is thrilling, and his emails are punctuated with exclamation marks. I can feel his excitement through the screen. I read and re-read his messages, watch a video he sends me of a cold night in the tent, and I wish that I could see the brilliant northern lights he describes so beautifully. When I go to bed, I pretend I am in the tent with him. Anything to avoid thinking about my pregnancy.

Joey returns home a week later, his cheeks ruddy from the outdoors, and I beg him to tell me every detail, like our son will one day ask for more stories before bed. ("One more, Mama," Teddy will say, after I've already told him four. So I tell him about superheroes and the Three Little Bears, stories I make up about him and his friends. He listens intently, wanting to stay up always just a few more minutes, and when I leave the room, I can hear him tell the stories to himself in his crib.)

I remember the details of Joey's trip as though I were with him and not miles away at home. I can feel the rocks slip beneath my feet on a razor-thin edge of a mountain I have never seen and I can hear the roar of the waterfall that signifies the end of the hike. I am trying to escape my own reality, my week at home forgotten, and my memory is filled with the details of a trip I never took.

WHEN I AM FOUR AND A HALF MONTHS PREGNANT, I SIGN UP for a prenatal class being held by a doula at a local hipster baby store. I want to allow myself to consider the possibility that this baby could survive. It is early fall and the days are still bright when Joey and I arrive at our class early on a Saturday morning. We sit in a circle and I look at the other couples sitting around the room. I feel foolish. The women are many months further along in their pregnancy than I am. When we go around the room, introducing ourselves and sharing our due dates, I feel my armpits dampen when I share my own. I am envious of their big round bellies and I long to be as pregnant as they are. I sit through the morning in a haze of shame.

When we leave the class for lunch, Joey and I are arguing loudly, about what I can no longer recall, but Joey is confounded by my sudden outbursts toward him. We walk the streets, scouring restaurants for anything I will agree to eating, and I walk one pace ahead of him the entire time. I feel so insecure for coming to this class because I know the risk of losing my baby is still high, that all of this could end in an instant, and I am taking it out on Joey.

Two weeks ago, at an appointment with Dr. Comeau, she listed all the possible complications based on the faultiness of my womb. Even though my baby was now past the twelve-week mark, I wasn't given much hope. "You could lose the baby at any point; your baby might not be able to grow properly; you are at a high risk for a preterm delivery, and even if you make it full-term, your baby could be breech, rendering the need for an emergency C-section."

I considered how unlikely it was to go well.

"All right," I replied, feigning bravery to myself and my doctor, because what else could I do?

When I am sitting in that prenatal class with all of the smiling, pregnant women, I don't feel like I am one of them. I jut out my stomach in an attempt to look more pregnant than I am, trying to fall in step with their conversations about wishing for a "natural delivery" because they all agree our bodies will *just know what to do*. I smile and agree with them even though I know my body has no clue what the fuck it's doing.

During the second day of class, the doula hands out sheets of paper that include instructions on how to create your own personal "birth plan." She recommends we make copies of our plan and hand it to the admitting staff on the labour and delivery ward. It is all so certain. I look at the women eagerly discussing what they want to do when they have their babies. I am still living in the world of *if*. I want to belong to the "birth plan" club where you ask for certain songs to be played in the delivery room or ice chips to be made into tiny stars. I want to talk with these women about having children like they are a sure thing. When I get home later that day, I throw away every handout the doula gave us. I put on my miscarriage outfit and I sit on the couch, waiting for my baby's heart to stop beating.

As my pregnancy continues, I feel the taps from our baby inside, a gentle and insistent reminder that they are still alive. These taps plant a seed of hope for the life I am carrying, and I cautiously plan for the arrival of our baby. I rearrange our spare room into a nursery, and I buy a onesie with the words *Worth the Wait* scrawled in childlike text over an image of a turtle. I outgrow all of my pants and I enjoy buying the ugly maternity clothes that fit my ever-expanding belly and thighs. I am filled with pride when a co-worker tells me one day, "Oh wow, you can really tell you're pregnant," because it all means my baby is still alive.

I can feel my body changing each day. Suddenly, I can smell even the subtlest of scents from across a room. Pregnancy turns me more bloodhound than woman. I can smell the hint of mint tea from across a dining room potently, its scent lingering in my nostrils the way I used to smell a roommate's cologne before a night out. Its offensive scent hung thick in the air, lingering long after he left for the pub. My enhanced sense of smell deters me from foods I normally love. As a coffee lover, I am startled when the scent of fresh coffee brewing churns my stomach instantly. I recoil at anything not deep-fried or salty. The thing I crave most is orange juice. I drink large, cold glasses greedily each morning and afternoon. It quenches my thirst in a way not even sports drinks could during the rigorous soccer games I played when I was a child. It feels to me more like the jump in the lake after the game that cooled my body wholly.

I've never had a good sense of my body. I bang my hips on the edges of tables and stub my toes on the corner of our bed constantly, bruises forming on my legs and arms. I feel as though I lack the ability to see my body as it truly is. In university, I spent time with a nineteen-year-old woman, Melissa, who had Down Syndrome. During one of our afternoons together, we had to walk across campus to a coffee shop. Melissa left her coat in her mom's car so I took off my jacket, handing it to her. She tried to put her arm through a sleeve, but it didn't fit. I tried helping her, but the jacket wouldn't budge. In my confusion, I realized that for the weeks we'd spent together I had seen myself as older than her, more mature, bigger. But none of this was true. We were only two years apart; she was an adult, and her body was fuller than mine. I blinked, finally seeing clearly, and we walked closely together to go for coffee, my jacket flapping behind us, draped across our shoulders like a blanket.

As my pregnancy progresses, my body awareness dwindles and I am like a baby calf, banging my body on the sides of doorways and trying to fit in places my body no longer can. I am out at a dinner one evening and I need to shuffle past my friends to get to the bathroom. I stand, trying to squeeze between the wall and their shoved-in chairs, but I realize I cannot suck in my stomach to move past them, my belly has grown too large, and I feel like I did that day in university, confused by my utter lack of self-awareness. It is only now that I can see how pregnant I have become.

To try and ease my anxiety, I use a hand-held Doppler, a miniature version of the technology used during ultrasounds, throughout my pregnancy to listen to my baby's heartbeat. I squeeze store-bought lubricant onto my stomach, mirroring what my doctors do, and I place the probe against my skin. The machine is the same size as the Walkman I carried around as a girl, and the probe looks like a child's microphone. When I switch the knob to the "on" position, the static is always piercing. I move the probe around my rounded stomach, pushing hard against my skin as I try to find the heartbeat. I close my eyes, listening for the *whoosh*, needing complete focus to catch the first beat. Once I hear it, I am flooded with relief. The sound reminds me of the ocean, comforting and rhythmic, except it's not entirely like the sounds you hear when walking along the beach. The sound is separate from the thing itself, as though I am holding a seashell to my ear, trying to feel the tide at my feet, trying to will my baby into being. I hold the wand steady with one hand and turn up the volume with the other. I listen for a moment, comforted by the *whooshwhooshwhoosh* of my baby's heart. Numbers flash on the screen: 135; 157; 140. I keep a record of the baby's heartbeat. A string of numbers that looks like a message in need of decoding. The message that my baby is still alive.

I never tell Joey how often I listen to the heartbeat, how often I need it to soothe my anxiety. It feels shameful that I can't ease my worries on my own. I take the device to work, tucking it into my bag still filled with pads in case I start bleeding again. I slide it into my scrubs' pocket during my breaks, and listen to its reassuring sounds in the bathroom. I wake during the night and slip into the baby's room, closing the door silently behind me. I sit on the rocking chair that I will one day rock my son in, and I listen to his heartbeat while I try to calm my own. I pack the Doppler when I visit friends or family, using it as often as—or perhaps more than—a toothbrush. I want to know the moment my baby's heart stops beating. I want to listen in case it slows. I imagine racing to the hospital and demanding help to save my unborn baby. I want control, and I fool myself into thinking this is it.

I AM TWENTY WEEKS PREGNANT, AND AFTER WEEKS OF REGULAR ultrasounds, I go in for my scheduled in-depth scan. This ultrasound is reminiscent of what is seen on TV and movies, rather than the internal scans I have grown accustomed to. My belly is round and large, and I feel truly pregnant. After settling onto the table and greeting the now familiar tech, Joey and I get to see our baby in their entirety. We see their miniature heart, its four beautiful chambers beating in synchronicity.

We watch as our baby flips and turns around in my uterus, performing acrobatics, making the tech say, "You've got an active little one in there!"

She asks if we want to find out the sex. We both shake our heads no. We have no desire to ruin the surprise of finding out. A moment we both speak about with such anticipation. The moment that Joey is still so certain will come.

After the scan is complete, we leave with a photo in our hand of our baby tucked inside. The contours of their nose and bow-shaped lips are beautiful. I hold on tightly to the photo the whole drive home.

I AM AT WORK TWO DAYS AFTER OUR SCAN AND MY CELLPHONE rings. It is my OB-GYN. After saying hello, I excuse myself to the break room to talk.

"We found something on the ultrasound that is a bit concerning," she says, her voice professional and emotionless. I sit on the brown couch and look up at the microwave that always displays the wrong time. Fixing my eyes to the red numbers, I let them go blurry as I brace for what's coming.

"We noticed your baby's kidneys have what's called hydro-nephrosis. There is a slight swelling in each of them, making them bigger than they should be. Alone, that wouldn't cause us to worry, but we also noticed your baby has a second marker on their scan."

Marker. The word used in the medical field, and in my profes-sional life, to describe the risk for a genetic condition, one that can be potentially life-threatening. It is typical for babies to have at least one, as bodies develop in all sorts of different ways, but two or more puts a baby at higher risk for a genetic anomaly. My baby has two.

"The second marker we found is in your baby's brain," my doctor continues. "They have what's called a choroid plexus cyst. A pocket of fluid—likely cerebrospinal fluid—located in the middle of their brain. Normally, if a baby has just one of these markers we wouldn't be concerned. With two, however, we need to do more testing to look for possible conditions. Your baby is at higher risk for having an abnormal set of chromosomes. Based on the two markers we found, we need to look for Trisomy 18 and Trisomy 21."

I slump over the coffee table and put my head on my arms, my belly pushing against my thighs. I turn on speakerphone while she explains what will come next. A detailed blood test, a more in-depth ultrasound, and possibly an amniocentesis, an invasive procedure in which amniotic fluid is removed from the uterus for testing.

Due to my work in pediatrics, I have an intimate knowledge of these conditions. Trisomy 21—Down Syndrome—is familiar to most, but Trisomy 18 makes my heart skip a beat. Babies with the unlucky duplication of the eighteenth chromosome have a life expectancy that is impossibly short, usually less than a year, and one that is often riddled with hospitalizations. When I was first pregnant, Joey and I had discussed the possibility we might have a child with a disability. We claimed we would welcome any child wholly, without condition, but we conveniently forgot the adoption checklist we had completed only months earlier.

When applying for adoption, each couple must complete a grim checklist of physical or intellectual conditions they are willing to accept in their adopted child. It is an unnatural act that forces you to put conditions on what is intended to be an unconditional love. Our adoption checklist demonstrates that we were not as generous as we always thought we'd be. We were not, in fact, willing to adopt any child when given the choice. We were selective on our application, saying yes to things like Down Syndrome and cleft palate, but leaving blank the selection for severe cardiac defects or global developmental delay. If I could not control the outcome of my pregnancies, I could at least control what my adopted child's life would look like.

This isn't like our adoption checklist, though. This is biology and genetics, two things I cannot exert my will upon. I can't say yes to Down Syndrome and no to Trisomy 18. I can't say I only want a child if they will survive and outlive me. I can only receive what is coming and not even my doctor can tell me what it is I will have to accept.

I hang up the phone after writing down the dates for my next series of tests; they will start the following day. I go back to the unit in a daze, trying to focus on work rather than what my doctor has just told me.

My manager pulls me aside. "Is everything all right?" she asks gently. "You seem off."

I am comforted that she noticed, and I tell her everything. She asks me if I want to go home, to take the day to rest, but I tell her I need the distraction of work to make it through the day.

I call Joey on my next break. Pacing this time in the small break room instead of sitting on the well-worn brown couches, I walk around the coffee table in circles, occasionally banging my knee on its edge. I tell Joey everything I know. He keeps reassuring me that everything is going to be fine, but I can hear through his reassurances that he is scared, too.

Joey and I are holding each other's hands tightly when we arrive for my appointment. We are on the special ultrasound floor, where they have higher-resolution imaging and fancy computers that measure the length of every single body part within only a tiny margin of error. The technology is intended to catch every marker possible, providing statistics and predicting outcomes. I feel like we are going to see a fortune teller when a nurse pulls the curtain back and we are beckoned to come inside.

I grew up having my fortune told by my great-aunt Bessie. She practiced tasseography—the art of reading tea leaves—and during many of our trips to my grandparents' house, Bessie would visit and tell our fortunes after supper. She had bright, unnaturally red hair and her laughter would ring throughout the house, making even a mundane family supper feel like a party. I loved when she visited. She would be seated or standing at the head of the table as she instructed us to drink our tea and gently swirl the leaves that remained on the bottom of the cup. One by one, we carefully handed her our delicate teacups, nervous about what she would see—even though our futures, according to her, were always bright. The many gold bracelets on her wrists jingled pleasantly as she turned our cups over and over in her hands, and we listened intently as she told us what she saw.

I am longing for Bessie's fortune-telling when Dr. Smyth walks into the room. She has short curly hair, mostly grey with traces of light brown remaining, wire-rimmed glasses, and a subtle pink lipstick. She smiles warmly and shakes both of our hands.

"I'm going to be taking a lot of pictures," she says. "You can watch on the screen up here." She points to a monitor high up on the wall, nearly touching the ceiling. "And I will explain everything I am doing. I will tell you exactly what I find as I go."

Her assurances that we will receive answers in real time is comforting. Having a doctor instead of a tech perform the test means we won't have to wait. Time is of the essence on this ultrasound floor, since markers can be life-threatening. She squirts the warm jelly onto my stomach, and we watch as she takes her time examining our baby's body.

"Here is your baby's brain," she says as her wand rotates slightly on my stomach. "You can see the cyst right here." She pauses a moment and I hear the click of photos being taken. We see a large bubble in the middle of our baby's brain. It is obvious even to us.

I inhale sharply as she explores the neck fold and spinal cord.

"It all looks good."

I exhale.

"Here's your baby's heart." The doctor taps a few buttons on the computer, and we see red and blue flash across the screen as our baby's heart pumps rhythmically. She turns a knob and we listen to the ocean-like *whoosh* of our baby's circulation. I close my eyes for a minute, listening to the sound I am so accustomed to hearing.

"The heart looks perfect."

I open my eyes and smile.

"All right, if you two don't want to know the sex of your baby, I suggest you look away while I scan their kidneys."

Joey and I look away from the monitor. After a few minutes, she tells us to look back as she fills the screen with a still image of two kidneys. They look like the silver bean necklace I wear around my neck. She uses the mouse to draw lines across each tiny organ, a red number displaying its diametre.

"The right kidney is a bit bigger than the left. But the left is really close to being normal-sized. It's reassuring to know both kidneys are not severely impacted."

I'm relieved with every word she says.

The doctor measures our baby's femur and counts digits. Ten fingers, ten toes. She takes the probe off my stomach and the screen goes black. She's done, but she needs to run more calculations on the computer before she can tell us more. She sits at a second computer in the corner of the exam room and we watch from the bed, looking over her shoulder, as she measures our baby's skull and looks more closely at their brain. When she is done, she turns her chair around and smiles.

"Good news, folks. Your baby seems to only have those two markers, the cyst and the swollen kidneys. Everything else looks great." She smiles broadly, appearing joyful with her prognosis. Perhaps these scans are unusual for her and she normally has the task of telling people, just like us, that their baby has more issues than they originally thought. I think of the doctors who had to give me bad news in the past and it feels ecstatic to be on the other side this time.

"That's great, thank you." I smile at Joey who squeezes my hand. "So, you don't think they are at risk for any genetic condition?" I need to hear her say out loud that our child will be born, and that they will be born healthy. I am begging the fortune teller to hand me my future with a certainty nobody, not even Great-Aunt Bessie, can give.

"No, I don't think they are at an increased risk. In fact, you don't need an amniocentesis because your risk remains quite low and the test comes with its own risks."

I get off the bed and after we thank her, she puts her hand on my shoulder and says, "Try to relax. Your baby looks fine."

I repeat her words over in my head, trying to ease my worries, trying to believe what she said is true. But later that night, before going to bed, I turn on the Doppler and listen to my baby's heartbeat. *Whooshwhooshwhoosh.*

11

▼

THE DAYS TURN SHORTER AND COLDER, AND MY ANTICIPATION for the winter mounts. My due date is in late February, and our baby's arrival will be a bright spot in the middle of the darkest season. I imagine bringing our baby home bundled against the cold and settling into our new life as a family of three. I don't flinch when Dr. Comeau tells me, at twenty-eight weeks pregnant, that I will need a scheduled C-section. My baby is breech and has run out of room to turn around. *Bring it on*, I think. I have long forgotten my desire to plan a "natural birth" with all of my fellow mothers-to-be from the prenatal class. I have only one thing on my imaginary birth plan: please let my baby live.

I relax a little with every week that ticks by, and soon enough Christmas is upon us. Joey and I begin to talk with more certainty about our baby's arrival now that I am almost seven months pregnant. We plan to prepare our bags for the hospital after the holidays and I picture the outfit I want to wear and the music I plan to have playing when we welcome our child. I am working over Christmas this year and the children's hospital is always festive during the holidays. Santa visits children confined to hospital beds, brightly coloured decorations line the sterile hallways, and the intensive care has its own artificial Christmas tree that we decorate during a quiet night shift. Even though I'll miss being home with Joey and my family, I am looking forward to my shifts spent with my colleagues and patients.

After my twelve-hour shift on Christmas Eve, I come home to a candlelit dinner, and Joey and I open our stockings. I put on my pajamas and we settle on the couch to watch a Christmas movie. I fall asleep almost instantly with my head on Joey's shoulder. Shift work is becoming more and more difficult the larger I grow, and I am always so tired at the end of the day. I have only been asleep for a few minutes when I suddenly jump off the couch. I look at my soaked-through pants and run to the bathroom.

Joey, startled by my sudden dash out of the room, follows closely behind and keeps asking, "What's wrong? Jo, what's wrong?"

Deep breaths punctuate each word as I say out loud what I instinctively know is happening. "My water broke. The baby's coming."

I get changed and Joey runs around the house, gathering things we might need. He packs both of our toothbrushes and nothing else. When we discover this, hours later, we laugh at how that it is the first, and only thing, he thought to grab. While we walk to the car though, our breath like two ghosts in the dark, we are both so scared we can barely speak.

Joey scrapes the frost off our windshield. When he sits down in the driver's seat, he rubs his bare hands together, holding them against the heater for a moment. While we drive down the road, we pass homes lit up for the holidays while Christmas music plays on the radio. I call my mom.

"Joanne, how many weeks are you?" my mom calmly asks me.

"Thirty-one," I reply.

"Exactly," she says, and I can hear the smile in her voice. "You're in your third trimester. The baby is going to be okay." She is calm and she repeats this to me one more time before I hang up. Her words are exactly what I need to hear.

I had been counting down the weeks during my pregnancy until I reached thirty. I knew that after thirty weeks' gestation, the likelihood my baby will survive increases dramatically. My friends knew this too, and they celebrated my thirtieth week with a cupcake that said *30!* and took a picture of me smiling with it resting on my belly. I didn't know when they snapped the photo that I'd be racing to the hospital a week later.

When we arrive at the registration desk, my pants are soaked through again and the woman behind the counter asks me to calm down and explain what is happening more slowly. I inhale, explaining our situation for the second time.

The woman is typing as I speak. She pauses briefly and says, "So, what you're saying is, you think your water broke?" She looks at me with skepticism in her eyes.

I look at my sopping wet pants, resisting the urge to shout at her. I reply as calmly as I can, "My water *has* broken." I had learned by now that, as a woman, I would often be dismissed, as though I didn't know what was happening in my own body.

We ride the incredibly slow elevator to the fifth floor where we wait in the prenatal-assessment unit for the resident to come in. A few days earlier, I had been sitting in this same room being assessed for Braxton-Hicks contractions that had been unusually strong. I came in to be checked before my Christmas shifts at work to be sure nothing was wrong. I was told by the resident that day that there was a ninety-nine percent chance I would not go into labour in the next two weeks. I left the clinic, relieved with the prognosis of another two weeks of pregnancy.

That same resident who had seen me days earlier is my doctor again on Christmas Eve.

"Well," she says, smiling. "I guess I was wrong."

I try to smile back.

After several minutes of checking and re-checking, I am told that yes, my water had in fact broken (not that I had had any doubt), but I am not in labour. The resident explains how the contractions I am having are not powerful enough to jump-start my body into delivering my baby. They are reactionary, she says, likely in response to my water breaking. They are considered blips, practice contractions, barely strong enough to be captured by the monitors attached to my belly. She expects they will stop in a matter of hours. I am skeptical because my body feels as though it's ready for a delivery, but I sit back in the stretcher, trying to believe what she is telling me, that maybe my baby won't be born so early after all. My body insists otherwise.

Minutes after my doctor's declaration of labour not being imminent, a contraction emanates from the most central place in my body, like the core of the earth or the pit of a cherry. It sends waves of pain outward, hitting my spine and twisting back around my stomach. I feel like I am a dishtowel being rung out. The clench releases and my body relaxes. The monitors that could barely register my practice contractions begin to alarm. A second tightening comes, stronger, more insistent than the last. My mouth makes the shape of a small O, my breath exhaling without sound. My world shrinks as if I am entering a tunnel, every bit of my attention turning inward. My nurse comes into the room quickly and she looks intently at the long sheets of paper printing from the machine, landing ribbon-like on the floor below. I place my hands on my swollen belly and the truth of what I've known since I leapt off the couch is reinforced.

I am in labour.

My nurse yells out the door for the doctor to come back.

The resident rushes into the room, looking at the pages the nurse is pointing at and then at me, more sheepish this time, and says, "Well, I think you are out to prove me wrong, aren't you?"

A second nurse comes into the room and rolls me onto my left side. A needle full of steroids intended to expedite the maturation of my baby's lungs is jammed into my bum cheek. The burning liquid feels as though I have been branded with a red-hot iron and I call out in pain. A third nurse arrives, and the team wheels me briskly from the assessment room into the birth unit. Joey is carrying our winter coats and half-jogging beside the stretcher.

My care is handed over to a new team and my nurse explains how they are going to try and slow my contractions medically. They want to stall the birth, but I need to prepare for the arrival of a baby who wants to be born. The clock rolls past midnight and it is Christmas day. I cling to the siderails of the bed as my contractions come in frequent, painful bursts, watching my knuckles whiten with effort. Every fifteen minutes, my nurse gives me a handful of pills and she sits patiently beside me, waiting to see if they will work.

As it nears five in the morning, my body begins to relax in response to the medication. The contractions slow to a dull hum rather than a loud roar, as though a rough sea has suddenly turned docile. Joey's eyes start to close; he appears exhausted in the chair beside my bed and I snap at him to stay awake. Mumbling about needing to get food, he wanders out of our room and into the vacant hallway to look for something to eat—or more likely, a reprieve from his snarling wife.

When Joey reaches the nurses' desk, he asks them where he can get a snack. The nurses take pity on him and one of them goes out back for a minute. Working the night shift on Christmas Eve means lots of food to share, and she fills a paper plate with treats, sending him back to our room. When he returns, he holds up his festive plate, grinning ear to ear. He sits in the armchair beside my bed and begins to eat a shortbread cookie when he pauses, remembering I'm not allowed to eat anything.

"Should I go eat this outside?" he asks, cookie held in mid-air.

"No." I smile. "I want you to stay here with me."

A little before seven in the morning, having averted an early Christmas morning delivery, we are taken to a room on the seventh floor where I am told I will live until our baby is born. They claim this could be hours, days, or even weeks, but I don't believe my baby will stay put that long. I pray for enough time to receive the second shot of steroids, the medication that will allow their lungs to be in the best possible condition for an untimely birth.

Joey and I doze off and on for a couple of hours before we call our families.

"You guys have the worst luck," my brother-in-law says when he comes on the speakerphone.

"It would be boring if it went any other way!" I say lightheartedly. We hang up after wishing each other a Merry Christmas and I sit silently in my hospital bed. My smile fades as I look out the frosted window, running my hands over my belly, encouraging my baby to stay put.

On Christmas night, my family crams into the hospital room and we eat turkey brought in Tupperware containers and open presents. Wrapping paper litters the floor and my nurse pretends she doesn't notice the abundance of guests filling my room. My large family far exceeds the visitor limit, but she winks at me and closes my door after handing me my pills, leaving us to spend the evening together. The kindness I am surrounded with makes me weepy.

My parents perch on the cot that is made up for Joey, my brothers fill the only chairs we can find, and my sister and Joey sit on the bed with me. We laugh and play games, as though we are all sitting around a Christmas tree. Even though I am exhausted, it is a relief from the intensity of the day we've just had. After they leave, my nurse comes back in, strapping the monitor to my swollen belly, and I get to hear the reassuring *whoosh* of a heartbeat before trying to fall asleep. As I close my eyes, I am overcome with gratitude that my baby is still inside.

My nurse wakes me in the middle of the night. She apologizes, but it's time for my second shot of steroids, and after I roll over displaying my naked bottom, she quickly pushes the plunger on the needle. The white-hot flash of pain makes my eyes sting and I arch my back as my body reacts forcefully, trying to escape the needle's torture. The nurse removes the needle swiftly, placing the palms of her hands on my skin and applying pressure, an attempt to provide me with some relief.

Two more nights pass in a blur, and I am still pregnant. I am adjusting to life on strict bedrest and am allowed to sit in a wheelchair for thirty minutes a day. I spend these minutes washing my hair, which is now a permanent rat's nest from lying in bed. I have a scheduled ultrasound each morning and I love being able to see my baby so frequently. It calms me. And that morning, when the doctor pauses on my baby's face, we see them blink twice and their eyes open wide as if they know they are on camera. The room goes silent in awe. They look around and we see them take in their surroundings, the whites of their eyes visible behind small black irises. It is in this moment that I can see my baby is full of life, their eyes providing me a glimpse of who they will one day become. They appear gentle and curious as they gaze upon the inside of my womb and I feel hopeful for my future as their mother. I now finally believe that I will one day look into those eyes without a screen obstructing my view, catching glimpses of mischief and happiness, sorrow and pain. It is this moment, when I gaze into the eyes of my unborn child, that I will recall moments before they are born, summoning the belief that everything is going to be okay. I want to put my hand against the screen as if they can see me; I want to touch their face, coo to them softly, encouraging them to stay put for as long as they possibly can. I want them to feel me, to know that I will do anything to keep them safe. The silence of the room is interrupted by the click of photos being taken on the ultrasound machine, capturing the moment I first locked eyes with my child.

"You never get to see that," the doctor says quietly, and I can hear the wonder in his voice. Our baby, who has miraculously survived despite all odds, never ceases to amaze.

I savour these last days of pregnancy in the way I enjoy most things when they are about to end. As a long-distance runner in my teen years, nothing felt better than when I turned the corner and the finish line came into view. A euphoria would strike when only seconds before, the burning of my lungs and muscles had felt overbearingly painful. I signed up for race after race not looking for a place on the podium but chasing the feeling of that moment. In the safety of this hospital room, in a building I know so well from my work as a pediatric nurse, I am enjoying my pregnancy more than I did in all the months prior. I know that being here will offer my baby the best possible hope of making it. It's as though I can sustain whatever pain I am feeling because I can see the finish line ahead. I can now imagine the moment my baby will be in my arms with a certainty I have never felt before, making each day more bearable than the last.

On our fourth day in the hospital, a neonatologist comes to visit us. He is part of the team in the Neonatal Intensive Care Unit (NICU) where our baby will be rushed immediately after delivery. I am sitting in bed, sweating profusely. Not because I am anxious, but because the steroids make me sweat like I've run a marathon, even though I've barely moved beyond the confines of my bed. The doctor walks into my room and after shaking our hands, he crosses his arms in an attempt to warm himself. I have insisted on opening all of the windows in our room and Joey is sitting at my bedside with his winter coat on, fully zipped.

"So, your baby might arrive at any moment," the doctor starts. "Or they may stay put until you are full-term. We have no way of knowing. If you progress back into full labour, I will not allow you to labour for long because your baby is still breech and small. We worry that if you start to dilate, it will not take much for the baby to come out."

I want to make a joke about the tightness of my vagina, but Joey's look of concern prompts me to stay quiet.

"I looked at your ultrasounds," the doctor continues. "Your baby appears to be in great shape even though there is not much amniotic fluid around them. You really broke your water, didn't you?"

"I do like to excel," I reply with a smile, trying to shatter the seriousness of his visit.

He ignores my comment and continues. "Your baby is small, though, and not only when compared to full-term babies. They are under the tenth percentile for weight of babies the same gestation, which is concerning. What we typically see with smaller babies like yours is they will need a bit more medical support."

My lightheartedness melts away because I know where this is going. I have been a part of many talks like this as a pediatric nurse. The "preparation talk" for parents on how they need to expect the worst. I feel sick because I can now read between the lines of his seemingly casual pop-in and I finally register the concern on his face.

"Your baby will likely need life support, a breathing tube, and to be put on a ventilator to help them breathe." The doctor looks at Joey to make sure he understands. He had obviously read the bold *MOM IS A NURSE* I assume is plastered all over my chart because any time I meet a new member of my health-care team, they ask me what kind of a nurse I am.

"Okay," I tell the neonatologist. "We can prepare for that." I sound braver than I feel.

He continues with a number of other scary side effects of being born too early—kidney problems, brain bleeds, feeding issues—but I can't grasp what he is saying anymore. I am picturing my baby connected to a ventilator, a scene I have been privy to hundreds of times as an intensive-care nurse, and it chills me more than the December wind blowing in through my windows.

The neonatologist finishes his speech and says, "I hope we don't cross paths again too soon," and he leaves. Joey and I sit in silence for a few minutes, letting the news sink in. He curls up beside me in the uncomfortable hospital bed, placing his hand on my belly. With a certainty we never felt during my entire pregnancy, we begin to discuss possible names for our baby. We don't know if we are having a boy or a girl and hadn't narrowed down our list of names before my water broke. Now, with a seemingly infinite amount of time in this hospital room, we try to give our unborn child their name.

Joey is looking at names on his phone and we are discussing the possibility of Oliver or Elliott if we have a boy, when Joey looks up and asks, "What do you think of Theodore?" I think for a moment and I agree that I love it too. Joey loves nicknames, and he comments how Theodore comes with a seemingly endless amount—Theo, Teddy, Ted—we love them all.

My contractions grow stronger and more frequent that afternoon, and my nurse comes in often to check on me. I feel a change in my body, and when my contractions hit five minutes apart, the resident is called in.

"Well, Joanne," the resident says, standing and removing her blue gloves, "you are three centimetres dilated and it's baby time.

I'm calling the OR. It's time to go for an emergency C-section."

My nurse instructs me to sit in a wheelchair while Joey frantically packs all of the things we have strewn about the room our short time there. We look at each other when we are alone for a minute and I tell Joey in a moment of honest fear, "I am not ready for this." I shake my head, trying not to cry, and I finally admit how scared I am.

Joey bends down and gives me a hug. He puts his hands on my shoulders, touching his forehead to mine, and says, "We can do this, love." He has given me this pep talk many times over the course of our relationship. His infallible belief that we can tackle anything together gives me confidence when I need it the most. I remember I'm not alone, that he's in this too, and his words reinstate my bravery as I lean my head against his.

My nurse reappears at the doorway to our room. "Time to go," she says, and she wheels me out into the hallway.

Once I am in the delivery suite, the room that holds an incubator and the familiar life-saving equipment from my life as a nurse, my contractions progress until they are only two minutes apart. I am breathing heavily, trying to remember anything from that long-forgotten prenatal class.

My doctor looks at me with concern and says, "Your labour is moving quickly, we have to get that baby out. I'll see you in a minute."

He leaves to prepare the OR and a moment later, another doctor pops his head into my room. He is an anesthesiologist I remember working with when he was a resident. He is now a staff physician and I smile, saying, "Jon, it's so good to see you." I pause for a moment and he gives me time to get through the pain.

"I want to make sure you're okay that I am going to be your anesthesiologist. I'm on call," Jon explains. He wants to make sure I am comfortable with him seeing me naked.

"Oh gosh, yes, of course," I reply, having long given up any desire for privacy as my contractions intensify. He introduces himself to Joey and then leaves the room. Joey laughs and says I am like a VIP since I know so many of the people caring for us. I am comforted by Jon's familiar presence and I know he will not be fazed by whatever he is about to see, even though it does involve much of my exposed body.

I am walked into the OR and two nurses help me step onto the flat bed. It is similar to the ORs I've seen in the past: metal stirrups at the foot, monitors, doctors and nurses walking briskly around the room. It's cold, and I shiver when my nurse opens my gown in the back and instructs me to bend forward, curving my spine like a rainbow. She holds my hands and counts out loud, while Jon expertly slides a needle into my spine, giving me my epidural. I count to twenty in my head and try to forget I am about to lose all feeling from my chest down, and the surgery I am about to have while fully awake. I lie down on the stretcher and look up at the ceiling. It is brushed metal and I can see hazy outlines of the activity below. I am now in the hands of the team assembled at my bedside and I feel a calmness wash over me. I no longer feel afraid. I am simply existing, my body no longer under my own care, and instead of feeling helpless I feel relieved. For the first time in months I relinquish my desire for control, and I breathe easily.

In, out. In, out.

The monitor beeps with my heartrate and Joey is perched by my head on a stool, dressed in full OR attire, mirroring the uniform of everyone buzzing around me. He smiles down at me and I shiver as the anesthesia kicks in, my body convulsing involuntarily.

My nurse wraps a warm blanket across my chest. "That will go away," she says reassuringly, and she pats my arm.

"I'm sorry to make you stay late," I say. It is now after seven and my nurse has stayed past her shift to follow me into the OR. "It wasn't my intent to have this baby at shift change." I smile, trying to be the nurse once again.

"Don't you even worry about that," she replies, and I see her eyes crinkle as she smiles behind her mask.

I close my eyes for a moment with Joey holding my hand and

I hear a voice say, "Joanne? I'm here!" I open my eyes, sitting in an awkward half-crunch since I am only able to lift my head off the table, and I see my co-worker Emily. She is waving from behind the curtain that has been erected at my chest, intended to keep my incision hidden from view.

I smile when I see her and say, "I'm so happy it's you!" She is part of the neonatal resuscitation team that has arrived to provide my baby with life-saving care. It is reassuring to know the people who are going to help my baby, even though Emily's presence reminds me just how precarious my baby's condition might be.

"All right, Joanne, are you ready to have this baby?" My surgeon looks over the drapes and I nod my head without pause. I feel strong, fearless. I am no longer feigning bravery. I am ready.

"One last guess from Mom and Dad—boy or girl?"

"Girl," Joey says.

"Boy," I say.

We look at each other and Joey squeezes my hand tightly.

"Well, we're about to find out who is right."

"Scalpel," he says, holding out his hand, and he bows his head to make the first cut.

12

▼

"Was the birth of your son traumatic?" Heather asks during our fourth session together.

"No, not at all!" I reply emphatically with a shake of my head, indicating how ridiculous her question is. My son was born, he was born alive, so how could it have been traumatic?

Heather is silent, and even after weeks of seeing her I ramble to fill the uncomfortable void. I'm sure it's the first lesson in psychology and I fall for it every time. "I mean, my water broke at seven months and I had an emergency C-section, but no, it was not traumatic."

Heather takes a couple of notes and our time is up.

With my surgeon bent over the lower part of my body, I wait anxiously for the moment my baby will be born. I feel tugging and lifting, and Jon keeps checking in with me.

"Almost there," he says, peering over the drape to where I can't see. "I see two little feet."

Feet! Two of them! I am elated my baby has feet.

After only a couple of minutes, the surgeon lifts my scrawny little baby like when Rafiki holds up Simba in *The Lion King* and Joey announces in a voice filled with pride, "We have a boy!"

My son is screaming, his arms flailing, and I breathe a sigh of relief at his intense screams. His arms are outstretched as the doctor shows him to me above the curtain, and I've never seen anything more beautiful. The neonatal team takes him from the surgeon's hands, taking him beyond my view, which is shrouded by cords and drapes. I lift my head off the pillow, trying to catch sight of him, but he's gone to the people who I know will keep him safe. I am relieved that Joey follows to the other side of the room, but I wish I could jump off the table and join them both. It feels unnatural that my baby is no longer inside me, and even a few feet away feels too far. His cries are reassuring though, and I lay my head back on my pillow to enjoy the moment of my child's birth. I hear Joey being asked if he'd like to cut our son's (*our son's!*) umbilical cord. I am smiling, listening to the sounds of my new family when his cries stop. The room goes silent.

Craning my neck to try and see what is going on, I turn to Jon who is still near my head and I ask, "Is everything okay?" Fear sweeps over me in the first wave of worry that is now meant for a person, my baby, not the hope of one.

Jon takes a step to the side, looking over the shoulders of the team caring for my son. When he looks back at me, he is smiling. "They are deciding which hat he should wear; he is fine."

My nurse asks if I'd like to hold him. "Yes, yes!" I answer enthusiastically—*would anyone have ever said no?*—and it is a gift that most mothers of premature babies are not granted. Preemies often need to be rushed away immediately to receive life-saving care.

When the nurse carries my son to my chest, placing his tiny body beneath my chin, I feel the sum of every fragment of joy I've ever felt wash over me like a wave. An elation I never knew could exist fills my body and radiates warmth like a warm spring day after a long winter. I feel somehow more alive than ever before, as though I, too, have just been born. Tears pool in the crease of my neck before I realize I am crying.

I strain to see my son's face. He is covered in warm blankets and a hat conceals most of his head, an attempt to protect his vulnerable body from hypothermia. His face is turned toward me, resting just below my chin, and I catch glimpses of a cheek, dark eyes, and a nose. I kiss a hand with fingernails that look like tiny white seashells and I love him instantly. I feel fully and wholly changed. I had gone into that room a woman, and when my son is placed on my chest, I became a mother. I am his mother.

After a brief moment of being able to hold my newborn son,

the nurse tells me she has to take him to NICU. He needs to be assessed and settled into an incubator. My tender-hearted husband doesn't hesitate when they ask him to take off his scrub top and sit in a wheelchair, to cradle our three-pound son against his skin for the transport to NICU. Normally, this is a task reserved for new mothers, but in an emergency delivery such as ours, the father is sometimes asked if he is willing to provide the body-heat a premature baby so desperately needs. I am unable to see the nurses place our son on Joey's bare chest since the surgeons are still working on piecing me back together, but Joey later tells me that in those few moments alone with our son, he was filled with immense pride and love for the baby he longed for as well. He cradles him protectively against his chest, the nurses covering them both in heated blankets, and gazes down lovingly while the two of them are wheeled through the back hallways of the OR. He recounts those moments as a gift he would have never received if things had gone differently.

Our son has been born alive, and he is healthy enough to be cradled by each of us in his first few minutes of life.

TEDDY LOVES TO HEAR THE STORY OF HIS BIRTH. "TELL ME I WAS a born, Mama," he pleads, usually before bed. I am used to the familiar way he adds or drops words accidentally, but the meaning is never lost. I have the story perfected, making him the hero every time. I start with, "It was Christmas Eve…" and I tell him how I leapt off the couch, telling Daddy, "This baby is going to be born!"

I tell him about the Christmas lights we saw as we raced down the cold road to the hospital and how a doctor told us, "This baby can't be born on Christmas!"

He giggles at the voice I use for the doctor.

"Why?" Teddy asks, and I tell him how he needed to have his own special day.

I explain how we waited four long days until finally another announcement, spoken in a booming voice: "This baby will be born today!" I replay the moment the doctor pulls him from my belly, holding him in the air, and we both sing the first lines of the "Circle of Life." I tell him how he comes out screaming and strong and how when I see him for the first time, his knitted hat tickling my chin, it is like watching the most incredible sunrise you could imagine. I tell him how he is the most beautiful baby I have ever seen.

I tell Teddy how he needed a spaceship to get bigger and how he spent weeks beneath bright purple lights. He loves the colour purple. He asks about the mask he had to wear, wanting to hear how he was a superhero without a cape. I tell him how we sang to him, cuddled him, and that the second-best day of our lives was the day we got to bring him home. The version I tell him is full of poetry. How his eyes were as dark as midnight and his ears as soft as velvet. His cries were like music, his little voice the crescendo of our lives.

When the story ends, with the happy family of three coming home together, he almost always says, "Tell me again, Mama."

I repeat the tale to my son until he is mouthing the well-rehearsed words, knowing where to pause, waiting expectantly with a smile on his face for the moment we break into song. My re-telling of this story is slowly changing my memory of the day. Rearranging it until I start to see it through the eyes of my son. The day of his birth. The day he joined us, screaming to let us know he was alive, and how euphoric I felt. In this version, there is no mother breathing deeply to calm her nerves before a surgeon pulls her son from her body two months early. There is no pain from pregnancies that came before or after. There is no stress or guilt or shame. There is only one thing that fills this version from beginning to end: joy.

In the recovery room after my C-section, I wait anxiously to be given permission to go to my son's bedside. To pass the time, Joey and I call our families to share our news.

"A boy!" we cry on speakerphone, and we hear the cheers erupting from everyone we tell.

An hour later, I am wheeled in my stretcher into the Neonatal Intensive Care Unit (NICU), my freezing not entirely worn off, for the first time as a mother and not as a nurse. I watch as the nurse lifts my son out of his incubator, all of his cords and wires getting tangled in the process, and expertly places him against me. It is a move I have performed many times myself as a nurse, yet it still amazes me how they are able to get him into my arms so safely. I stroke my son's head, inhaling his sweet scent, and I never want to leave him again.

Teddy was breech for most of my pregnancy, his head remaining upright, and I pictured him standing, like a baby in a Jolly Jumper, while his feet tap danced on my cervix. He often stretched when he was inside, and I could feel the strain beneath my skin as he arched his back and pushed his head forward. My heart-shaped womb provided little room for him to move around, and when he did this, my stomach contorted into an elongated shape and I could see the clear outline of his skull. I would put my hand over his head in those moments, cupping it in my palm, giving it a gentle rub to say hello.

When I am holding him in NICU that first night, his head fits entirely in my palm and my fingers wrap over his forehead like bangs. My arms have to overlap in order to cradle him, his impossibly small body fitting in my forearm, and he looks like a doll. I close my eyes, feeling the top of his head as though he is still inside me and stretching. I run my fingers over the spot on his head where the pieces of his skull haven't yet fused, and I know he is mine. I recognize him instantly.

I open my eyes and look at my son. "It was you all along, wasn't it?" I whisper.

After being allowed to hold him for the first time, I am taken to the postpartum floor, the place where babies typically sleep in clear bassinets beside their mothers, but my baby stays behind, two floors away. The distance feels vast, and I am acutely aware of our separation. I catch a few hours of sleep with Joey in a cot beside me and the moment I open my eyes I wake Joey, telling him I am going to NICU. I need to get back to my son. Joey rubs his eyes, exhausted, but I am already standing, waiting impatiently for him to follow. I have expertly unplugged my IV pump and hung my catheter on the handle, acting as my own nurse.

As I walk toward the door, my nurse appears in the doorway and asks, "Where are you going?"

"I'm going to NICU," I say, trying to walk past her.

"Well, I need to do your morning assessment and you have to take your meds," she says, blocking my way. I begrudgingly return to my bed while she pushes on my fresh incision, assessing for any signs of excess bleeding, while I inhale sharply from the pain. When she is done, I stand and start to walk down the hallway once more.

I see my surgeon walking toward me and he stops me in the hallway.

"Joanne," he says. "I can't believe you're walking already." He smiles broadly, holding my chart in his hands.

"Yup, I am heading to NICU," I say for the second time, continuing to walk down the hall, away from my room and him.

"I need to do a morning check on you," he says, gesturing to my empty hospital room.

I impatiently follow him back to my room, giving curt answers to his post-operative questions, and I nearly run out the door the second he is done. "If anyone else tries to talk to me," I say to Joey, who is in step beside me, "I'm not stopping." He smiles in response and puts his arm around my shoulders as we take the elevator to see our son.

That morning, I sit at my son's bedside, cradling him against me. His three pounds of weight feel heavy with meaning. He has light fuzz covering his shoulders, dark blue eyes that are often closed, and small white dots, milia, speckled across his nose like the ghosts of freckles. I kiss those dots over and over until one day they disappear quickly, and without warning. A metaphor for his infancy, I think. His dark newborn hair will also disappear months later, leaving his head more bowling ball than peach fuzz. When his hair grows back, a shock of curls will appear, which I lovingly coil around my fingers. When he turns one, I cut a single, perfect ringlet that I tuck inside his baby book to keep.

A group of medical personnel approaches our bedside and the charge nurse explains it is time for morning rounds. Well versed in the process of medical rounds, I sit taller in my chair, anticipating the full report on my son's health and the medical plan for the day. I look around and recognize colleagues and acquaintances whom I have run into on many occasions over the last several years of working in the same building. I smile proudly while holding my baby and I wave at those I know like a celebrity of sorts. People smile back even though I am certain they are shocked by my haggard postpartum appearance.

The nurse practitioner provides a report on my obstetrical history, which I learn is customary when a baby is first born; it will provide helpful context to those caring for my son, to know how he came to be born so early.

"Mom is a thirty-year-old Gravida 3, Para 1, with a history of two prior miscarriages, a bicornuate uterus, endometriosis, fibroids, a subchorionic hematoma…" She stops suddenly before continuing with her report, which includes the early rupture of my membranes and the status of my son when he was born, looks at me, and says, "Wow, you are so lucky to have him."

It feels like my heart stops beating then, because she has put into words exactly what I have been feeling since I laid eyes on my son. I cannot believe my luck. I am still in shock that he is here. That I am a mom. That I am *his* mom. The tubes, the alarms, the UV lights, everything else disappears when I see him. I can only see the manifestation of everything I have ever wanted. For years I had been holding my breath while trying to will this child into life, and when she says those few words aloud, I am finally able to exhale.

DURING MY FIRST AFTERNOON WITH TEDDY, HIS NURSE presents me with a triangle of fabric made from a baby blanket. It feels soft and new, exactly like the receiving blankets I had bought for his arrival, the ones still sitting idly at home, unopened. I am told its purpose is to encourage bonding between Teddy and me while he is in NICU. For the nights when I have to sleep two floors away from where he lies sleeping in his incubator, alone.

The nurse holds up the little baggie that encases a pink triangle of fabric. She looks apologetic. "I'm sorry, we don't have any boy colours left."

I smile back, shrugging my shoulders. "That's okay. He's a modern man."

I look at my son as he sleeps in his incubator, his hands laced behind his head as though he is a grandfather asleep in his favourite chair. I don't intend to raise my child with strict gender norms; he is growing up in a generation that will hopefully value equality more than mine. One that will allow people to be who they are outside the confines of their biological sex. My plan is to allow him to simply be who he is.

Teddy's third Halloween recently passed. The first one where he was able to provide input into his costume. The years before, I dressed him in poorly made animal costumes, a sheep and a dalmatian, taking dozens of photos of him alongside pumpkins and piles of leaves. This year, though, he could participate.

To prepare him for the holiday, we buy books about trick-or-treating, a Halloween party, and children dressing in costumes. I point to the costumes and say, "Look, Teddy. You can be anything you want to be." He looks seriously at the photo, studying it intently, and points to the sister in the book.

"I want to be a princess," he says, requesting a purple dress just like the girl in the book.

"That's a great idea, buddy!"

We purchase a sparkly, purple princess dress for our son to wear the following week. Joey helps him into the dress on Halloween night, letting him step into it gracefully, and then presses the Velcro tabs, closing the back. I feel such love for my kind-hearted husband who loves his son without condition. Teddy spins around the house, showing off his dress, and we clap for him. We go trick-or-treating with our happy princess and I feel such joy that we are able to provide our son this moment of innocent happiness without having him feel any judgment or restriction in expressing himself.

Back in NICU, the nurse explains to me that to help Mom and baby bond—*I am Mom, I remind myself*—I can tuck the pink fabric into my shirt, allowing it to soak up my scent. It will be placed inside his incubator, allowing him to smell me even when I'm not nearby.

"It's amazing, the power of scent," she explains further. "We see babies calm down instantly when the triangle is moved close to them, and we have seen their vitals improve, too."

I diligently tuck the fabric into my shirt, hoping to give my son his first security blanket for the couple of hours a day I have to spend away from him.

When it is time for me to go back to my room, I pull the triangle out of my shirt, smoothing out the now-wrinkled fabric. I reach into the incubator and place it over Teddy's eyes like a rudimentary sleep mask, trying to remind him he has a mother. I watch his monitor for a few minutes and when his heartbeat drops a few beats, I pretend it is because of that triangle. Each time I return to his bedside, I love seeing this little scrap of fabric the nurses have lovingly placed in the incubator as they cared for him in my absence. I see it tucked across his chest, underneath his head, or resting on his forehead like a fainting cloth.

I perform my own ritual to feel close to my baby when I have to sleep so far away. I grab a bundle of his blankets and one of the hats he wears daily and steal them away to my room. With my nose pressed against the fabric of his doll-sized hat and blankets, I fall asleep almost instantly. His scent in the fabric is like the earth itself, as though a hole had been recently dug in the soil, ready for a sapling to be planted. It is mixed with a sweetness that reminds me of the cinnamon buns my great-grandmother used to make. When I stir in my sleep, I cling to the fabric, bringing it to my nose and falling back asleep with the reminder of my baby pressed against me.

ON MY SECOND NIGHT OF MOTHERHOOD, I AM IN MY ROOM, floors away from Teddy, trying to get comfortable. After taking a sip of water, I inhale a tiny bit into my lungs and I have to cough. I realize with panic that I avoided taking any pain medication all day because it meant leaving my newborn son's bedside. I purposely ignored the nurses' requests that I take care of myself. I only wanted to care for my son. When they would call throughout the day, saying it was time to take my medication, I insisted I was fine since it meant leaving NICU. I didn't move beyond my chair beside Teddy until I was forced to go to bed. The surgery I endured is an afterthought compared to the intense love I have for my baby. With the anesthesia now completely worn off, however, it feels like if I cough my incision will rupture.

I half-cough and sputter, splinting my stomach with my arms wrapped tightly around my middle. The pressure needed to generate a cough feels like my stomach will split in two. I move onto all fours on the mattress, looking up at Joey who is standing by helplessly, asking me what's wrong.

"Nurse, please," I choke out, and Joey presses the call button.

I rock back and forth, shaking my head, trying to stop my body from doing what it needs to do to protect my lungs. In a moment of fatherly instinct, Joey thrusts the pile of baby blankets I had taken from NICU into my face.

"Smell this," he urges. I inhale deeply, stimulating a cough, and cry out in pain, clutching the blankets to provide some relief.

After taking a few breaths to steady myself, I sit back up and look with wonder at Joey. "How did you know to do that?" I ask, and he shrugs his shoulders. The power of our son's presence, even the hint of his smell, amazes us. It is a natural analgesic, relieving my pain and calming me instantly. We realize then just how much magic he brings to our lives already, how his delivery into this world has altered us in ways we will never be able to fully articulate.

I settle back into the bed, having taken the pills my nurse gave me for pain, and I curl up with my son's blankets. I also realize, then, that Joey and I now belong to each other in a way we never did before. Our son binds us tightly together forever. We love him more than anyone else possibly could. We know him intimately: he is a part of both of our bodies. We understand what it means to love someone else more than we could ever love each other.

When I think of potential accidents or catastrophes, being made to choose between Joey or Teddy, the choice is easy, even if the outcome would be anything but. And I know Joey will always choose our son over anyone else, including me. It's an unspoken rule that we will give anything to keep this child alive.

13

▼

TEDDY IS TOO PREMATURE TO BREASTFEED WHEN HE IS FIRST born. His stomach lacks the ability to digest milk, and his mouth is too uncoordinated for the task. Colostrum, the very first milk a mother produces, is filled with antibodies that are invaluable to a newborn, especially one as vulnerable as Teddy. I am instructed to pump my breasts to provide our son with the precious immunity the thin, milky fluid provides. During those first few days after his birth, I pump my breasts by hand, feeling entirely bovine, while Joey collects the tiny drops of colostrum into a syringe that is labelled and carefully handed to our nurse. The nurse then reaches into the incubator and squeezes a few drops into Teddy's mouth like a baby bird.

When Teddy is three days old, I begin producing breastmilk. When I hook myself up to the pump that day, I feel a rush of emotion as intense as the sensation in my breasts. It's something I've never felt before, as though a string is being pulled from my nipples. My breasts tingle and I cry inexplicably, not from pain, but from the overwhelming emotion as I look down at the bottles that are filling with the first of my milk. The hormones needed to produce breastmilk have created a rush of oxytocin and dopamine, and I am elated as the milk flows from my body. When the milk stops, I turn off the breast pump and the sound of its rhythmic whirring stops. I pull the plastic contraption from my chest and pour the milk into a single, one-ounce bottle. I hold it between my thumb and forefinger, and I start to laugh. My milk is a rich orange colour. I show the bottle to Joey and he laughs, too, saying, "Maybe you drank too much orange juice, love." I wipe my tears, the high of producing the first of my milk dissipating, and I label the bottle proudly, snapping a picture before carrying it to the nurse.

I AM SITTING ON THE STOOL BESIDE MY SON'S INCUBATOR ONE afternoon when a co-worker, Tim, comes to say hello. Tim is the friend at work I can always laugh with. Although our work, caring for sick children, can be heavy, I always feel lighter for having spent time with him. I admire his skills and we can always count on the other to tell a joke at just the right time to ease the tension. A sense of humour is an unspoken, even necessary, skill to survive as a nurse.

Postpartum has been unusually unkind to me. I know I look terrible. The fluid given to me during surgery has pooled in my neck and feet, but Tim looks at me with such kindness it is easy to imagine we are talking as we always do, beside a patient's bedside. Except this time, the patient is my son, and I am the anxious parent. How strange to be on the other side of the bed. To watch as everyone gathers around and talks lab values and plans. I am desperate to feel a sense of normalcy, and when I look down and see my stomach hanging over my legs, I grab the flab and I ask Tim, "When do you think they're going to take out his twin?" I am desperate for Tim to play along, to pretend that it's business as usual.

His laughter lights up the curtained-off area around us with the vibrancy I need. Most people would have said "Oh you look great!" which I know is a complete lie. I still look fully pregnant and I need recognition of the sorry state of my body.

"You do have a bit of a gut on ya!" Tim says, and it is the kindest thing anyone had said to me all day. Tim stays to chat with me for a few more minutes, and before he leaves, he pats me on the arm, telling me to hang in there.

A doctor I work with also comes to visit. After he asks how I'm doing, he assumes a stance I have seen dozens of times: his tie is tucked in between the buttons of his shirt and his hands are on the small of his back, the tips of his fingers sliding into the top of his grey dress pants. He leans over the incubator and watches my sleeping baby for a minute. His face remains neutral while he scans my son's body. He turns, looking closely at the monitor that displays Teddy's vital signs—his heart rate, breathing rate, blood pressure—they are numbers I am familiar with and have studied endlessly since my days as a nursing student. They are invaluable sources of information, providing insight into the inner workings of a body, and as a nurse I diligently watch for any subtle changes that tell me a patient may be getting worse. It is often this doctor, the one now standing at my son's bedside, who I would call when a patient's vitals told me something was wrong. He silently watches the numbers scroll by, and I look carefully for any signs of concern that might flash across his face. It's as though waiting for him to give me an order like the nurse I still am, but he turns back to where I am sitting and smiles. I exhale with relief, and he says, "Well, he looks pretty good, doesn't he?"

"Do you think he's okay?" I need so much reassurance, and I will take whatever I can.

"He looks great." We speak for a few minutes before he returns to his office.

My eyes fill with tears when another co-worker, Lauren, shows up one evening. We have grown close over recent months, our babies sharing the same due date. We used to call them *the twins* and we spoke about our pregnancy woes while working night shifts and performing the physical labour of health care. When Lauren walks up that night and peers at Teddy in his incubator, her belly is large, and I know she is picturing her own baby because I am, too. She tells me how when she found out Teddy had been born already, she couldn't believe it. I place my hand on her stomach, telling her baby to stay put, and I can see how emotional she is. When her daughter is born two months later, on time and without complication, I celebrate the arrival of Teddy's twin and imagine how things could have been different had Teddy been born then, too.

Before delivering, I was nervous to be so exposed in my workplace. To have a child is an extremely intimate thing. Your body is on display and you are vulnerable. In those days after delivery,

I don't recognize my body when I look in the mirror. My breasts are leaking, my legs are swollen, and my belly is round, as if Teddy had yet to be born. And yet, I find myself grateful to be surrounded by my caring co-workers.

The kindness continues as the days pass in NICU. I always have someone to talk to at two in the morning when I wake to check on my son. I receive hugs and laughs when I pass people in the hallway. I am seen in my worst state, but instead of feeling exposed, I feel loved in my vulnerability. I am comforted by my co-workers' presence at my bedside; they are looking out for me, and keeping an eye on my son in the moments I can't be there. It keeps me sane during those weeks in the windowless NICU.

After being discharged from the postpartum floor, days after Teddy's birth, Joey and I were checked into the Ronald McDonald House, a charitable housing option for families of sick children. It is down the hall from NICU, allowing us to stay close to our son. It has a large common area with soft couches and chairs where our family and friends will congregate in the weeks to come. Our private room has two twin beds and a wooden nightstand with a lamp sitting atop its glossy surface that gives off a soft yellow glow. It, too, is another series of windowless rooms, and the persistent lack of natural light further distorts our concept of time. Over the weeks to come, days bleed into nights like drops of ink into water. The only demarcation of time is when, during morning rounds, we are reminded of how many days it's been since Teddy's birth. We have access to a shower and a washer and dryer, necessities that now feel luxurious while we are marooned within the walls of the hospital. We are vulnerable, unable to control much, and to stay in a warm, comfortable environment brings calm to our never-ending days.

We run into other parents in the hallways and common areas at all hours. It is normal to pass another parent at two or three in the morning delivering bottles of milk, worried looks on tired faces. We smile at each other quietly, often keeping to ourselves. We become friendly with with a couple whose baby is in the crib beside our son. Their original due date was within days of ours. They are well-accustomed in life in NICU, though, as their son was born at 24 weeks, a whole seven weeks before Teddy made his appearance. We eat dinners together, the four of us sharing stories about life in the hospital, and when their son passes NICU milestones—his first day without oxygen, his ability to eat from a bottle—we cheer along with them, as they do, us.

Teddy spends much of his time in a clear incubator and is bathed under bright purple lights to treat jaundice, a condition that turns his skin a ruddy tone and the whites of his eyes yellow. He wears a purple felt mask to protect his eyes from the harsh light, and when the nurses take it off, the skin beneath remains a slightly different hue. It looks as though he has been inside a tanning bed. When I spend hours holding him, I watch his skin turn from its natural pink to a deep bronze, like the Edgar Degas sculpture *Little Dancer of Fourteen Years*.

When I was a girl, my mom hung a print of the Degas painting *The Dancing Class* above my bed. In the centre of the painting, depicting a late-nineteenth-century ballet class, a ballerina makes eye contact with the viewer. She is smirking, as though she has a secret. I always loved that look in her eye. She looks strong and defiant, traits I admired in others from an early age. I always felt meek, less sure of myself, wishing to be liked by everyone. I remember standing on my tiptoes on the bed, my nose nearly touching the painting's glass frame. I dreamt of being a ballerina as a girl and the painting, and the girl at its centre, filled my heart with a desire I knew would never be realized.

"STRAIGHTEN UP," MY BALLET TEACHER SAYS TO ME. I AM WEARING a pale blue leotard, white tights, and soft pink ballet slippers that are somehow always untied. The outfit highlights my adorable toddler shape: a protruding belly and stubby, thick legs. I don't show much promise of becoming a ballerina and I will only take classes for a few months. Even at four, my teacher can likely tell that my body will never blossom into the elegant, long-stemmed flower it needs to be, for me to become a true ballerina.

I pull back my shoulders in response. She walks around the room, nodding to some of the girls, but she pauses behind me. She puts her hands on my shoulders, turning me sideways to face the floor-to-ceiling mirror. The soles of my slippers squeak against the shiny hardwood floor as I pivot in place, and the scent of new leather fills the air. She runs her hand down the curve of my spine, showing me my poor form.

"You have a banana back," she states, and with a tsk, she walks away. I try standing up taller, but I only push my stomach out further, turning even more banana than ballerina.

Years later, before moving to Edmonton with Joey, I search for adult ballet classes online, feeling inspired by my move to a new city. I picture myself attending classes, practicing for hours, and becoming a woman who is sure herself, like the ballerina from my painting. Someone who always does what is best for her, who cares more about her inner voice than the voices around her. Except I am the woman who followed her boyfriend to a city where she has no interest in living. I feel out of focus, a blurry outline of a woman, not at all like the powerful dancer in my painting who is brought to life by the dabs of pink on her cheek and the perfect arch of her eyebrow. I have dreams, most of which, I admit, are traditional, but I am more concerned with who I want to be *with* at this moment in my life than who I want to *be*. I want my boyfriend to turn into my husband and to have children with him. Beyond that, I am unsure of anything.

Moving to Edmonton felt like a chance to become the idyllic version of myself, to grow into a self-reliant, confident woman. And yet, by our second year of living in Edmonton, I have never attended a single ballet class and I have not managed to reinvent myself. Only my postal code has changed, but even that is impermanent. Joey remains the only thing I am certain of.

When a travelling Degas exhibit comes to the Alberta Art Gallery, I go to see it on my own. There I stand, in the wide-open gallery, staring at the bronze Degas sculpture in person. I want to reach out and touch the dancer's ballet slipper. Her toes are inches from where I stand beside the pedestal beneath her. I look at her in silence, feeling my back straighten.

Years later, as I hold my son in NICU, I stroke his impossibly small feet and I feel a stirring in my heart, as though every dream I've ever had is possible because he has survived. Maybe I'm not the woman I imagined I'd become—self-assured, opinionated, defiant—but I'm his mother, and that is even better.

TEDDY'S INCUBATOR HAS FOUR PORTHOLES, TWO ON EACH SIDE, allowing Joey and I to reach our hands inside and touch his delicate skin. I stroke the bottoms of his feet, loving how his toes fan outward instead of curling in. A primitive reflex that newborns have, and one that is delightful to watch. Even its name, the Babinski, is playful and sweet. He is hypotonic, his body lacking the muscle tone needed to curl into the tight newborn shape I am used to seeing. He is nothing like the babies who I've seen photographed as little balls wrapped in tightly wound cheesecloth. Without the walls of my uterus to constrain him, Teddy appears as though he is floating in water, his arms and legs splayed out like the tentacles of a squid. The nurses make him nests of blankets, filling his incubator with props that they tend to regularly. They are trying to simulate the resistance my womb should still be providing, but he is hard to contain, his arms and legs always finding a way out. He is thin and his skin is nearly translucent in places, dark blue veins creating a map across his body that I gently trace with my finger. He has cords and IV lines and his tiny diapers fit in the palm of my hand. I keep one as a reminder of his days in NICU, later adding it to Teddy's baby book. When I look at it now, it is unbelievable that we once had to roll down the top of the doll-sized diaper to fit his miniature hips.

One day, our nurse takes prints of Teddy's hands to surprise us, explaining how challenging it is to do so with full-term babies because their hands are always clenched in tiny fists. The hands of premature babies, though, are relaxed and open, providing us with another gift we would have never received otherwise.

I spend hours holding Teddy in the chair beside his incubator, unwilling to leave unless absolutely unnecessary. I don't want to lose a single minute with him. He mostly sleeps, and I read to him during the long hours we stay nearly motionless together. With our chests rising and falling in sync, as though he were still inside my body, I read him chapters of *The Great Gatsby*, allowing him to get used to the timbre of my voice, no longer muffled by skin and tissue. I read until I feel myself drifting to sleep, and I pass Teddy to Joey while I leave for a coffee and to pump milk.

The nurses are gentle with us, two new parents, and they encourage us to lift and care for Teddy as though he is not attached to so many cords and tubes. Joey, a man who has never before changed a diaper, is eager to partake in the physicality of fatherhood. When Teddy is not quite a day old, Joey rolls up his sleeves, our nurse instructing him what to do, and reaches into the portholes to change our son's diaper. He awkwardly pulls the soiled diaper out of the incubator, tossing it in the garbage. After he cleans Teddy's bum with the soft cotton wipes the hospital provides, neatly tucking all the cords back under the tab of his diaper, Joey turns to me and says, "I feel like this might be easier to do once we get home." I laugh in response, agreeing whole-heartedly, and feeling more in love with him than ever before.

On New Year's Eve, we visit Teddy's incubator just before midnight, settling into our blue armchairs to welcome the new year as a family of three. I watch his monitor, with its constant stream of numbers going past, waiting for the clock to hit 11:59. A nurse calls out a countdown, and the parents who are still awake join, counting down the seconds to midnight in unison. When the clock on Teddy's monitor strikes midnight, we hear a quiet wave of "Happy New Year!" ripple through the unit, barely above a whisper so as to not wake the babies who are asleep. Joey and I kiss Teddy's head. We have to take turns because he is so small. Joey and I then kiss each other, and my eyes fill with tears of gratitude. This year, 2017, was supposed to be the year we met our son, but how lucky we are to have him with us in this moment. To be granted extra time with my son is a gift I never expected. It is a gift, however, that comes with a cost.

14

▼

OUR DAYS DRONE ON WITH A SCHEDULE THAT CENTRES AROUND morning rounds, pumping breastmilk, and a number of other mundane tasks that make each day stretch on forever. While Teddy is unable to eat, an IV in his belly button, called an umbilical line, provides his body the nutrients it needs. I need to pump to trick my own body into thinking my baby is nursing. I have been instructed to pump every three hours, and I take this direction seriously.

I pump diligently to show my dedication as a mother. I set alarms on my phone to go off around the clock and when my alarm sounds, I excuse myself no matter what else is going on and retreat to either my son's bedside or my room to pump. I am anxious if I am ever on the verge of being even a few moments late. I go to bed around eight, and before turning off my light for the night, I check all the alarms I have set on my phone. Checking and re-checking them is the only way I can fall asleep.

My alarms blare throughout the night. After I am woken before midnight, I stumble my way into the unit to cuddle Teddy if he is awake. If he is sleeping, I gaze lovingly through the Plexiglas at his perfection. If my nurse isn't there, I leave my two bottles of milk on her desk, a precious gift for her to keep safe for my son, and I shuffle back to my room. Joey normally sleeps through my alarms since he is exhausted, not only from new fatherhood but from the hours he is still putting in at work, sending emails and taking calls while tucked away in common areas around the hospital.

I am living in a state of delirium, as all new parents do, and each night when I wake to my alarm, I pump, wash my supplies, and fall back to sleep. Sometimes I wake convinced I have missed a pumping session and frantically turn on the light to set up my kit, only to see two bottles labelled with the previous time, waiting to be delivered to NICU. I have dreams where I am attached to my pump and I try to pull the plastic off my chest, only to discover I'm not attached at all.

Around six in the morning after being in NICU for a little over a week, I wake to my phone going off loudly in our room. I reach to turn off my alarm so I can pump, but when I look at my phone, I see that it's NICU calling. With my heart racing, I answer.

"Hello?"

I am fully alert and filled with fear.

"We need you to come to the unit now," a voice says in a clipped tone.

"Coming." I hang up and turn to Joey who is still sleeping on the cot beside me, our two single beds making us feel more like siblings than husband and wife.

"Joe! Something's wrong. We have to go to NICU!"

Joey leaps from his bed and we scramble to put on slippers and pants, then race out of our room. It is this call that I've been expecting, dreading, since the moment we arrived to NICU. I have made plenty of those calls as a nurse, calls that wake parents from a restless sleep, urging them to come quickly because their child had gotten worse. I imagine all the horrible scenarios that could have caused our nurse to summon us and I am nauseous when we enter the unit.

We wash our hands as quickly as we can, up to the elbows as always, and as we round the corner Teddy's incubator comes into view. I am relieved that his bedside is not filled with doctors and nurses, the telltale sign something is seriously wrong, but the bright overhead light is turned on and Teddy's nurse is walking briskly around the room, gathering supplies. I search eagerly for the numbers on my son's monitor. All of his vital signs look good. I take a deep breath, hoping they called us by mistake.

"Thanks for coming," our nurse says when she sees us. "I'm worried Theodore is septic."

The word *septic* constricts my throat like I am being strangled by invisible hands. Sepsis, or septicemia, is an infection that spreads in the blood and can cause serious illness in anyone, but premature babies are most at risk due to their immature immune system. It can lead to multi-organ failure, life support, and in some cases, death. There are signs posted everywhere in NICU about the importance of handwashing and every time we enter the double-locked doors to the unit, we have to scrub our hands raw, up to the elbows, like surgeons, before being allowed near our son.

The fear of infection is palpable at every bedside. We have limited our son's contact with people during these precious early weeks, and even as his parents, we are instructed to avoid coming to NICU if we have even the smallest sign of a cold or flu. Anytime someone sneezes here, every parent goes tense, angrily searching the room for the culprit who dares spread germs near our fragile children. We spend hours daily scrubbing the space around our son's cot and I quickly and emphatically become a germaphobe.

The nurse explains why she is concerned. "I checked his stomach a half an hour ago, and he hadn't absorbed any of his food from the whole night. I had only been giving him one millilitre an hour and every drop was still in his belly. His belly is tight, and round, and I can see loops."

She points to Teddy's abdomen and Joey and I peer into the incubator. We watch as she gently touches his stomach, and we see it. His stomach looks as though it's filled with snakes writhing beneath his taut skin. His inability to absorb his food, being delivered by a feeding tube down his nose, and the tightness of his stomach could mean an infection in his gut.

"All of this can be a sign of NEC or sepsis, so I called the doctor. He wants me to draw bloodwork STAT to see what's going on. In the meantime, I have stopped all of his feeds and he is back on IV fluids."

I nod my head, familiar with the language she is using—I know that NEC means necrotizing enterocolitis, that it means the fragile tissue in Teddy's intestines could be inflamed. That his bowels could be deteriorating right in front of us, leading to perforation, infection, possibly death—but Joey looks bewildered. While the nurse gathers the rest of her phlebotomy supplies, I settle myself into the blue chair beside Teddy's incubator, preparing to hold him while he has his blood drawn. I translate the medical jargon for Joey while I sanitize my hands again, the squeak of the antiseptic bottle indicating it is nearly empty. I make a mental note to ask our nurse to bring more when this is over.

"They're worried he has an infection," I explain. "He could have NEC, which is when a part of the bowel dies, or he could have a blood infection." I say this using the calm disconnect I have adopted since becoming a nurse. I am back in survival mode and can't afford to become emotional. Joey's eyes widen at my explanation and he runs his hands through his hair nervously, peering at our son in the incubator.

Our nurse reappears and elegantly places Teddy in my arms, her well-trained hands navigating all of the cords and IV lines with ease. I stroke his forehead, giving him drops of sugar water to help ease the pain he is about to feel. My eyes scan his body, assessing him like I would a patient. After the nurse is done, we sit anxiously for the results.

An hour later, the doctor and the rest of the team arrives. This doctor is our favourite, his confidence and calm demeanour always welcome at our bedside. Joey grabs my hand, holding it tightly.

"I've been speaking with his nurse on and off since early this morning," he starts. "We were concerned about Theodore's belly, but the bloodwork results are reassuring." Joey and I squeeze each other's hands, our silent message that everything is going to be okay. "I'm going to assess his abdomen and see what's going on, but it might simply be that he isn't ready to eat yet." He puts his arms, with their expertly rolled sleeves, into the portholes of the incubator, and he pushes lightly on Teddy's belly. He takes his stethoscope out and places the bell on different parts of our son's stomach, listening intently with his eyes closed. When he is done, he takes an alcohol swab from his pocket and wipes his stethoscope in small, circular motions.

"Everything seems normal. I'm not too worried, but if he doesn't start eating food soon, we will have to look at putting in a more permanent IV line. That umbilical line needs to come out." He gestures toward the large plastic tube coming from our son's umbilical cord, the lifeline he's been attached to since birth. It is providing all the nutrients his tiny body needs, mimicking his life inside my womb.

The nurse practitioner on the team speaks up. "We should look at taking that out today. It's been in for almost twelve days."

The doctor thinks for a second. "You know what, he's doing well and has no signs of infection. Let's give him one more day. I have a feeling he's going to turn the corner. If his body doesn't learn to eat before tomorrow morning, we will put in a new line, but I think he's going to come around." The residents and nurses scratch their orders down, and Joey and I silently pray our baby will prove the doctor right.

Later that day, our nurse comes to see how Teddy is tolerating his food. She attaches an empty syringe to his feeding tube and pulls back gently to see how much milk remains in his stomach. The plunger barely budges, and it springs back into place when the nurse lets go. She smiles and turns to us. "It looks like he's finally eating." She looks down at our son and gives him a tiny head rub. "Good job, little buddy. Keep this up and you'll be out of here in no time." Joey and I look on proudly at our son's accomplishment, and I wonder if this is how I might feel when he one day graduates from high school.

The nurse triumphantly relays the message to the doctor when the team arrives for afternoon rounds, and we smile proudly during her report.

"Well," our favourite doctor says, "let's take that line out."

He leaves our bedside with his team trailing behind him, and Joey and I stand beside the incubator, caressing our son with our hands. We tell him how proud we are. "You just needed a little extra time, didn't you?" I coo. While I put my head on Joey's shoulder, I silently promise to always give my son however long he needs in life.

With Teddy now eating, his umbilical line removed, he is allowed to have a bath for the first time. Normally this occurs before two weeks of age, but things move slower in NICU. Our nurse wheels a plastic basin beside his incubator filled with warm water. We ask if we should strip him down and remove the cords and stickers that are stuck to his chest. She explains how pulling off the leads—the stickers and wires that monitor his heartbeat and breathing—can cause damage to his skin; it is thinner and more delicate than that of most newborns. Instead of peeling them off before the bath, she says we should bathe him with everything still attached. We'll let the warm water and gentle soap loosen the adhesive beneath, hoping to maintain the integrity of his precious skin.

I wrap Teddy in a towel before placing him in the water, at the instruction of my nurse. It feels odd to be swaddling him before he is wet, but his small size means he can't be exposed for long. We place him, towel and all, into the warm basin.

He is calm and serene when the water engulfs him. Tilting his head gently, I rinse water over his soft head like a priest performing a baptism. As I unwrap his towel, exposing his body to the water for the first time, he lets out a sigh. He loves it. I keep my hand protectively under his neck, and gently wash his body in an act that feels intimately maternal. His skin turns bright pink with every stroke of the cloth; even the softest of materials acts like an exfoliant against his premature skin. I gently pull off the stickers stuck to his chest and they leave angry welts in their wake despite my best efforts. He looks like a baby bird; a downy fuzz called lanugo covers his body, and it reminds me of how baby penguins fluff out their soft grey feathers after being born.

When the bath is over, I wrap him in warm blankets and towels. While cradling him, I tilt my nose toward his scalp, inhaling his freshly washed scent. He smells new, the way I remember babies smelling before I became a mother, and when I breathe in deeply, beyond the scent of baby shampoo and lotion I smell him, the sweet scent of my child.

When I bathe my son now, as a toddler, I still place my nose against his head and breathe in his perfect scent. The act of washing cannot erase the most beautiful smell in the world.

15

▼

Teddy stops breathing. In our weeks spent in NICU, his brain forgets to send his body the message to breathe. It is a side effect of being born too early. This happens often, sometimes several times an hour, and it is terrifying.

I watch with dilated pupils as my son's chest goes still and his skin turns from pink to white to blue. The numbers on his bedside monitor plummet to values that do not seem compatible with life. Numbers I have seen as a nurse. Numbers that cause me to lace my fingers together to perform CPR.

Joey and I stare helplessly at first, watching as the numbers rapidly approach zero, alarms blaring, with our nurse running to his bedside. They reach for him, taking him from my arms, or put their hands into his incubator to shake him gently. They scold him for being "a little troublemaker." Finally, he takes a big breath and his colour slowly returns, the numbers on his screen climbing back to normal. We watch this dozens of times and, with our nurse's encouragement, we learn how to intervene, to stir him to breathe on our own.

We are taught how to stimulate our baby. When he is in his incubator, I rap my knuckles against the Plexiglas as though he is a fish in a bowl. If I am holding him, I pull him out of the crook of my arm and lift him, shaking his shoulders gently or tapping the bottoms of his feet.

"Breathe, breathe, come on," I whisper into his velvety ears, glancing between him and his monitor for signs of life. There is always a moment of terror, a surge of adrenaline, until finally he opens his mouth and gasps like a guppy. His lifeless chest fills with air and his colour returns to normal.

I will look for the metronomic beat of his chest in the months and years that follow. I still look for it in our toddler. I imagine I always will. So afraid that I will one day find his chest still again.

Eventually, the nurses encourage us to let him recover on his own. "He can do it," they tell us. We watch, our hands ready, waiting for him to take a breath. I feel so much pride when his chest heaves and the numbers on his monitor return to normal. I will think of these early moments when our two-year-old son is learning to dress himself. A much lower-stakes exercise in allowing him to develop and become independent, but an act requiring patience and restraint on our part.

When Joey and I are alone with our baby behind the curtain, I am unable to stop myself from intervening. When our son turns blue, when I feel his body soften under the lack of oxygen, I involuntarily shake him gently or tap his feet. Joey, sitting beside me, looks at me as if to say, *You're not supposed to do that anymore,* but I can't resist my instinct to keep him alive. I won't.

IT TAKES SEVERAL WEEKS BEFORE TEDDY'S BRAIN LEARNS TO tell him to breathe regularly, and a few days before we are sent home, he stops turning blue and going limp in our arms. Teddy is nearly a month old now, still a month away from his due date, and with discharge becoming a certainty, I am forced to go home for a couple of hours to prepare for our son's homecoming.

I haven't left the hospital since my water broke over three weeks ago, and it feels unnatural to be driving twenty whole minutes away from Teddy. It is a sunny afternoon, rare for late January, but the air remains frigid and our walkway is filled with snow. I run quickly to get inside, stomping my boots on our entryway mat after I close the door behind me. Our house is mostly as we left it. Christmas decorations fill the living room and unopened red envelopes with holiday stamps sit in a neat pile on the edge of our dining room table. The air inside is stale, and it is eerily quiet; it has been empty since Christmas Eve.

A kind neighbour of ours, Jon, who noticed our sudden and prolonged absence, runs into Joey outside as he's unloading our bags from the car. He claps Joey on the back, congratulating him on the arrival of our son. Turns out Jon had been checking and re-checking our vacant driveway these past few weeks, scared something terrible had happened to us. Joey and Jon swap numbers, ensuring they will stay in touch, and we are comforted that he cares so much. It feels as though our son is already bringing us closer to our neighbours, providing us with a stronger sense of community just when we need it.

Joey and I spend two hours that afternoon scrambling to put away all of the Christmas decorations and washing every receiving blanket we own. I even wash the newborn baby clothes I bought months earlier, knowing they are far too big for my premature baby, who is still only five pounds. We planned to accomplish so much more—buy groceries, wash our own bedding, take a nap—but my mind is in NICU with Teddy. We are like two magnets and I am being pulled, drawn toward my son in a way that is overpowering and all-consuming. And I feel a connection to all mothers in this moment. During pregnancy, fetal cells cross the placenta and enter a mother's bloodstream. Those cells can lodge themselves into the tissue of a mother's body, where they divide and multiply, forever changing a mother's DNA. Even though Teddy has been born, parts of him still live inside me. Everything that passed between us when he was inside my womb persists in the urge to see him, hear him, and hold him in my arms. It's as though the bond between us only intensified the moment the umbilical cord was cut, his cells within me sounding an alarm only I can hear when he is far away. I can't ignore the pull of him any longer, I need to get back to my son. We drive back to the hospital and I am relieved to see Teddy's nurse holding him when we approach his bedside. He is okay.

And then, a little over four weeks after my son is born, I am sitting in the back seat of my car, with him bundled tightly against the late January cold. Tears roll down my face as I realize he is now fully ours. No more doctors or nurses or monitors, no more windowless rooms or days that feel endless. We are going home.

OUR FIRST NIGHT HOME IS RESTLESS. WE HAVE GROWN SO USED to the alarms and ambient noises of NICU that we never appreciated how *noisy* our baby is. In the quiet of our room, we hear him grunt and coo and make all sorts of noises we didn't hear in his first month of life. I jump at every sound only to discover our loudly grunting baby is sound asleep in his bassinet. As sleep deprived as I am the following morning, I am so happy to be home. The next day, Joey goes to the store to get all of the baby items we haven't yet bought. A bouncy chair, a playmat for Teddy to lie on, diapers and wipes. He leaves in the early afternoon and it is my first time completely alone with my son.

When Joey and I moved back to the East Coast, we spoke about buying our first home and we scoured listings, searching for the perfect house to grow a family. We toured a two-storey with tall maple trees lining the yard, an ocean view, and a park nearby. We walked upstairs, peering into a child's bedroom that had a crib in the corner. The walls were painted royal blue and a stained beige carpet covered the floor. They say to visualize your own life, your own things, when you're searching for a potential home. I could see our lives in this house so clearly. After we bought the house, I stripped the floor of the carpet, cutting my hands on the sharp staples, and Joey laid hardwood flooring that I softened with a plush rug. We painted the walls a mint green, setting up the room as a spare bedroom, but in our hearts, it was always our baby's room.

The night we took possession of our house, we packed a picnic basket and a bottle of wine. We used our new keys to unlock the front door, but it still felt like we were breaking in. Our footsteps and voices echoed off the bare walls around us and we laid a blanket where our dining table would soon sit. We ate sushi and drank wine from plastic cups, talking about all of our plans for making this house our home. After supper, we wandered into each room and I stood for a long time facing the big windows that stretch the length of our bedroom, staring at the ocean below. Joey came in behind me, putting his arms around my middle, and together, we soaked in the view that would become the backdrop of our lives.

We arranged our sparse furniture into the empty rooms, painted walls, and hung photos that we'd later take down and hang again in a new spot. I loved painting the baseboards a crisp white and I spontaneously decided to paint our living room a dark navy. I normally find dark colours claustrophobic and menacing, but the large windows that lined the north side of the room made it feel as though we were being embraced by a warm hug, rather than sitting in a cave. Our house became more of a home with every passing week.

During my first afternoon alone with Teddy, I look around our home, seeing it through fresh eyes. Everything feels as new as it did when we first moved in. I run my hands along our dining room table, picturing a high chair pulled in next to it and fingerpaint spattered on its wooden top. I walk upstairs, taking Teddy into the nursery, telling him that this room has been waiting for him for years. I go across the hall into our bedroom and sit on the bed looking out at the now-familiar scene below, made new. The trees that line our property are bare, giving an unobstructed view of the ocean. I am grateful that our son will grow up so close to the sea, and I hope that he will always feel at home next to the water. I carry him from room to room; I want to know what it feels like to mother him in each corner of our home.

I settle back onto the couch in our living room, the place we will spend many hours over the next several months, and I hold him tightly against my chest. The winter afternoon turns dark early, the sky changing from grey to a deep purple, and I stay in our darkened corner, quietly holding my son for hours. It feels as though a cocoon had wrapped itself around us, and I feel safe with him in my arms. "I need to remember this," I speak aloud into the silence of our home. I want to remind my future self, when early motherhood is only a memory, that these days were filled with long afternoons cradling my son, soaking up his infancy. I know his infanthood will be fleeting, and I need memories to cling to, reminding me I had cherished it all deeply.

Joey returns home, the front door blowing open, and I feel the chill of late January ripple through the house. He lugs all of the baby items inside and unloads them along with some groceries. I lean forward, planning to get off the couch to help, but Joey stops me, saying, "No, stay right where you are, Jo. I've got this. What would you like for supper?"

I sink back into the couch and smile as the smell of garlic and grilled chicken fills our home. Joey brings two plates into the living room and we eat perched at the coffee table. Joey cuts my food while I nurse Teddy. My husband smiles at me, placing his hand on our son's head, still in the crook of my arm, and we feel ourselves settle into our new life as a family of three.

I SPEND MOST OF THE NEXT FEW WEEKS CURLED UP ON MY couch with my son. He is most often in my arms, sleeping against my chest. My postpartum body is soft, my breasts full, and my stomach round, providing a comfortable place for Teddy to rest his head. I have mostly healed, although my body feels foreign, as though someone without an intimate knowledge of it has taken it apart and attempted to put it back together. A puzzle with pieces that have been forced into the wrong place.

Nerves around my C-section scar were permanently damaged during surgery, and the feeling has never returned. It left an area of my stomach feeling doughy to the touch, like my face felt after having a root canal when I was fifteen. I remember coming home after the painful dental procedure and touching my cheek and chin repeatedly while looking in the mirror. I had to see myself touching my face to believe I was making contact with my own skin. Parts of my stomach act the same way. As though part of my body remains ghost-like, othered, not quite me.

At night, Teddy sleeps in our bedroom in a wicker bassinet that we keep within arm's reach. Every morning, I wake to the sounds of seagulls, boats on the water, and the slight hum of traffic on the road. The sun creeps across my bedroom floor, casting a bright orange hue on the cool colours of the bedroom walls. Perhaps Mother Nature created sunrises as a gift to mothers. To be bathed in such warmth makes it hard to lament the hours of lost sleep. The moment Teddy stirs, before he has even opened his eyes, I am fully awake. I lift him from his bassinet, bringing him to my chest, and settle us both back into bed. I undo the clasp of my nursing bra and feed him, trying to get him back to sleep for a few more minutes of blissful rest with him in my arms.

When he can no longer be settled in bed by nursing, I bring Teddy's bassinet downstairs and set it on the coffee table, which is littered with baby bottles, empty coffee mugs, and soothers. He nurses often, needing to eat more than full-term babies do to gain weight. I give him iron supplements daily since premature babies do not have enough iron stores to ensure the healthy development of their brains. The medicine stains my clothes with what looks like rust when it dribbles out the sides of his mouth. He crinkles his nose when I slip the syringe of supplement into the side of his cheek, when he tastes the bitter medicine instead of the breastmilk he is expecting.

I drive Teddy twice a week to a new family doctor I am still getting to know. Dr. Comeau retired when I was five months pregnant. Shortly after passing my care to a new doctor, she called me unexpectedly.

"Joanne," she started, "would it be okay if I called in and checked in on how things go for you? I'd like to hear how your pregnancy turns out. If you agree, of course."

I was touched by her request, and surprised. *Perhaps she cared more than she ever let on*, I thought. "Of course," I replied. "Thank you for everything."

"I hope things go well for you. Take care, Joanne."

We ended the call and I reflected on our complicated relationship. It was difficult to reconcile the way I felt when she dismissed my concerns years ago and the conversation we'd just had. Maybe she wished she could have done more for me and perhaps had felt helpless in the face of my infertility. Maybe we were more alike than I realized.

With Teddy in his car seat, we drive to see our new doctor. A mirror is angled on the headrest so I can see his face in the rear-view mirror, and I check it constantly. I pull over every few minutes to place my hand on his chest, to make sure he is still breathing.

Our new doctor, Dr. Stewart, is younger than Dr. Comeau, and her British accent makes her seem friendly and warm. She looks like a music teacher with her frizzy blonde hair and collection of purple and bright red cardigans. She smiles every time she calls Teddy's name from the waiting room.

In her office, after helping me pull Teddy out of his car seat and onto the paper sheet, she chats with him while measuring his length. He cries, as being undressed in the cold exam room is a shock to his thin body, and his skin turns mottled. After the doctor weighs him on a metal scale I re-dress him, and he nurses while she asks how he is sleeping and if he is still spitting up after each feeding. Teddy is prone to reflux, a common ailment for those born too early, and the medicine he's been given to settle his stomach seems to be working.

Dr. Stewart hands me a yellow sticky note with the day's measurements. I will keep it in a box filled with other yellow squares that document my son's growth, and after standing to go to her next patient, she tells me I can stay as long as I need. Once Teddy is asleep, I pull him gently from my breast and bundle him back into his car seat. As we walk out, the receptionist peers at my sleeping baby and says, "See you in a couple days, little buddy."

Nursing a now five-pound baby at home takes much of my time. Teddy is a slow eater, getting sleepy when only half done, and I have to gently pull him off my breast, tickling his feet to encourage him to re-latch and eat fully. I learn how to nurse while doing other tasks around the house. I eat while he eats, wiping away crumbs that fall onto his head. I walk around my house with him latched, straightening pillows, smoothing the blankets on our bed. I learn to sip my coffee through a straw held at arm's length, so I don't risk spilling the hot liquid over him.

I keep an in-depth record of each feeding. How long Teddy spends latched on each breast and how often I change his diaper. I mirror what our nurses did in NICU—a form of record-keeping meant to keep him alive. The log is a mess of muddled numbers and incoherently scribbled times. I download a breastfeeding app with a timer made for this exact purpose, but I often fall asleep without remembering to turn it off.

My documentation of those early days is as inaccurate as my memory; it is clouded with a lack of sleep, and overwhelming love. What remains is a distorted version of what those days were actually like. I remember each one as a series of photographs, disjointed moments in time that I can sometimes string together, but which often stand alone. They feel like snapshots I can click through in my mind like slides on a projector. When I click fast enough, they play my favourite film.

I spread a thick blanket on the floor, putting toys and blocks and books on the bright fabric for Teddy to explore. We listen to music while the sun rises, casting a light across the living room. I sip coffee and watch him with enjoyment as his eyes take in what I have surrounded him with.

My friend is visiting, and I am trying to hold a conversation, but my head constantly turns to the bassinet, my eyes wandering to the clock. *He'll wake soon*, I think. Knowing my time without putting him to breast is limited, it is hard to stay focused.

We hang a Jolly Jumper from the doorway of our home. Its metal will scratch the molding from its overuse, and as soon as Teddy is strapped in the harness his legs kick excitedly. I lay a sheepskin rug on the floor beneath and dangle him above it, clicking the harness into the bungy cord above. He bounces, yelling with excitement, and seems to dance along to upbeat songs I play for him.

I get into the shower and I can hear Teddy's cries the moment I step beneath the warm water. I shower quickly, barely dry myself, and race out of the bathroom to soothe him. When I arrive, still wet, Joey is holding a sleeping infant in his arms. The cries were phantom, my brain creating distress when there is none.

There is so much laundry. Blankets, onesies, bibs, and clothes. After putting Teddy down for a nap, I carry a load to my basement, filling my washer with the bright colours and turning it on. I open the dryer and carry the still-warm bundle back to the living room. I fold each item into a tidy square. When Teddy outgrows each outfit, I place it neatly in one of the bins tucked away in a spare closet. Mementos of his infancy.

I pace the hardwood floors in Teddy's room late at night when he is fussy. My screaming two-month-old will not settle. Joey stumbles into the room to help and sees the desperation in my eyes. "Here, let me take him," he says, holding out his arms. I gratefully pass our red-faced infant to him and go back to bed, falling into a deep sleep that lasts only an hour before my son needs to eat again.

When Teddy outgrows his bassinet at four months old, I put him to rest in the crib down the hall that has remained empty for months. I pull the sheet taut against the mattress after laying him down gently, remembering the lessons I learned in nursing school. I leave the room only when I am confident there are no wrinkles—not even a slightest corner of a sheet—that could obstruct his breathing.

While he is napping, I remain vigilant. I periodically step into his room, pulling the sheet away from his face, and I count his respirations. It is an involuntary compulsion driven by my anxious new-mom state. When he wakes, Teddy's face is creaseless, and after picking him up in one arm, I run the palm of my other hand across the sheet, smoothing it, making it safe once again.

At nighttime, Teddy spends the first couple of hours in his crib, and the remainder of the night in our bed. We've heard all the evidence and advice against co-sleeping before, have been told cautionary tales of babies suffocating beneath blankets and sheets. And yet, nothing feels more natural than having my son tucked against me for the duration of the night. I love having his body pressed against mine, and we both sleep better beside each other. In my darker moments, I envision going to his crib and discovering him lifeless and blue. I decide that if it comes to that, I'd rather have him die in my arms.

Joey sometimes wakes before us, tiptoeing out of the room to shower and leave for work. He tells me later about how he sometimes stood at the doorway, watching us sleep. Teddy's small frame facing mine, my body curled protectively around him. It feels luxurious to wake up next to my baby. It is an intimacy I have never before experienced.

Well-intended family members and friends remark that rocking my baby to sleep, and holding him as often as I do, is spoiling him. My quick response to his cries is viewed, by some, as a failure on my part. I respond to my son at a moment's notice and I nurse him to sleep every night, holding him in the chair we bought for this exact purpose. I watch as his jaw slackens, and his mouth pulls away from my nipple. I tuck my breast back into my shirt as he drifts off to sleep. I stare at his beautiful face, the way his lips part slightly when he is first asleep, and I don't care what anyone has to say; I don't want to do anything but hold my child. I respond to my internal voice and let the words of others waft into thin air as soon as they are spoken aloud. I am learning to care more about my own voice, to trust in it, instead of those around me.

Teddy is a restless baby. He sleeps fitfully, grunting and jerking in a way that is characteristic of many premature babies. He tucks his legs up against his belly in response to the pain of his immature stomach, still learning how to digest. He wakes often to feed, and he moves constantly, always trying to get comfortable. But I find this soothes me. The moments he is still and quiet are too reminiscent of death. Like ultrasounds without the *whoosh* of a heartbeat. A still image instead of waving arms and legs. I check and re-check his crib when he's quiet, expecting, with my whole body, to find him dead. I place my hand on his quiet chest, counting his breaths, and I relax when I can hear the rhythmic sound. As a toddler, Teddy will continue to bang around in his sleep, forever flailing his limbs and pinging them off the rails of his crib. The gentle banging that I hear in the middle of the night allows me to roll over and fall back to sleep, knowing he is alive.

16

▼

WHEN TEDDY IS FOUR MONTHS OLD, WE TAKE HIM TO GERMANY. Joey is presenting at a conference and we plan the trip thoroughly, getting a passport for Teddy that will make us laugh even years later. When I take him to get his photo, he is fussy and only wants to nurse. He cries incessantly, and only when he pauses between sobs to inhale does the photographer snap a picture. His face is red and splotchy, and tears stain his grey sweater. Our angry newborn's mugshot.

Even though I have travelled quite a bit before this, I am still the notoriously bad packer I was as a child. When I was nine, my mother did most of my packing for my week-long summer camp. In an attempt to encourage my independence, she asked me to pack my bathing suit on my own. I had two, and I couldn't decide which one to bring. So I procrastinated. I played Barbies with my sister and rode my bike. The next day, an hour into the two-hour drive to camp, my mom asked me which bathing suit I'd packed, and I looked back at her with wide eyes. She chastised me, asking why I hadn't done what she'd asked. We drove up to the camp, where wooden bunks dotted across a field like bales of hay and the field overlooked the warm waters of the Northumberland Strait. When the counsellors announced it was time for a swim, I shamefully pulled on my soccer shorts and T-shirt, feeling out of place next to the frilly pink swimsuits of my peers. As I got older, I never learned the lesson my mom tried to teach me that summer. I forever pack at the last minute and I inevitably forget one important item each trip I take.

Having a newborn, however, means I need to be thoughtful about my packing, and I know I can't procrastinate. Weeks before the trip, I lay out suitcases and spend hours writing out lists of things we need for our week away, checking and re-checking them. As the day of our trip approaches, I feel satisfied that motherhood has made me a new type of traveller. One who thoughtfully plans and packs for her trip, one who will have everything they need when they arrive.

We land in Berlin and our suitcases do not. We wait, ask for assistance at the help desk, but decide we need to check in at our hotel before it gets too late. We take the bus with just our carry-on luggage and Teddy, who is strapped to my chest in the baby carrier. As soon as we check in to our hotel room, I nurse Teddy atop the crisp, white sheets. Joey opens the windows to let the fresh air of this new environment fill our room. I feel adventurous to have taken our small infant to a new country and I am eager to explore, but I wish my well-packed bags had arrived. It feels like a cruel twist of fate that the first time I thoughtfully pack them, they don't arrive as scheduled.

The next day, we check baggage claim and our luggage has still not arrived. The clothes I wore on the airplane feel grimy and full of sweat, and Joey is wondering how he will present at the conference in his T-shirt and jeans. Teddy is the only one unfazed by our situation. He happily wears the same onesie, cooing at our furrowed brows as we check and re-check the status of our bags. I turn my phone off in frustration and look over at Teddy who is shaking his rattle, kicking his legs in enjoyment. I pause, grinning at our baby living in the moment, and my frustration dissipates.

Our bags arrive two days later, just in time for Joey's pre-sentation. When he leaves in the morning, I strap Teddy to my front, filling a backpack with everything we'll need for the day. The two of us walk mile after mile along canals and cobblestone streets. I breastfeed him on a bench overlooking a courtyard decorated with graffiti and posters. I take him to the Berlin aquarium, where, while he mostly sleeps, his eyes widen with awe as he watches the jellyfish floating in the dark around us. In a children's toy store, I buy Teddy a wooden car that shoots across the floor when you pull back on its wheels. I picture the boy that I will one day play cars with as I place the small parcel in my bag. We visit Checkpoint Charlie and the Berlin Wall museum, where I learn how families were suddenly split apart by its overbearing presence. I bounce Teddy in his carrier when he gets fussy, unable to imagine our family being separated in such a way.

When we return home after our trip, I feel an overwhelming sense of accomplishment, as though I have discovered a new version of motherhood. A version where I can travel around the world with my son, relax, and enjoy my time with him without fear. Here, in this place, I am the kind of mother I have always wanted to be, the kind I had always thought I would become.

I REALIZE I HAVE POSTPARTUM ANXIETY WHEN TEDDY IS ELEVEN months old. I am settling into the rhythm of life with a child when the fog of new motherhood lifts, and I reflect on my early days with Teddy. My anxiety was likely born long before he was. I remember the complications of his pregnancy, my compulsive listening for his heartbeat, my fear when my water broke too soon. I think back to my first two pregnancies, and how they planted a seed of doubt for any pregnancies that would come after. Even though I only learn its name when Teddy is nearly one, my first conscious awareness of my postpartum anxiety comes one week after we bring Teddy home.

A nurse calls and I sit on the stairwell of my house, responding to her questions about breastfeeding. I have just spent a month in NICU receiving expert advice on nursing and I wait for her to ask how I am doing, so I can explain that I am terrified my son is going to stop breathing the moment I leave his side. I want to tell her how scared I am when it's stormy outside because the wind and snow that beat down on our windows and the waves that crash against the shore drown out the sounds of my newborn son's breathing. I want to tell her that in those moments, I curl up like a cat beside his bassinet at the foot of our bed so I can listen to him breathe. I want to tell her that I am so convinced

Teddy is going to die that I have trouble putting him down. That I feel my fight-or-flight instinct every moment of every day, that I can't let him out of my sight for even a few minutes. That if a friend or family member is holding him and I can't see his face, I am unable to sit still. That in those moments, I pace my kitchen, busy my hands with laundry, will myself to do anything but rip him out of their arms to make sure he is alive. I am convinced he would have died countless times over if I were not so vigilant.

When I am home alone with my son and need to get dressed while he is sleeping soundly in his bassinet downstairs, I race up and down between our living room and bedroom to make sure he is still breathing.

I run upstairs and pull on a pair of pants. Run back downstairs to check.

Breath.

Run upstairs and pull on my socks. Run back downstairs.

Breath.

I convince myself that this is how everyone experiences motherhood because nobody asks me if I lie on the hardwood floor for hours some nights, my hand on my son's chest, certain that it will stop filling with oxygen at any moment. Nobody asks me if I have to pull off to the side of the road thirty times on a four-kilometre drive to check my son for signs of life. Or whether I start to leave our house an hour early, knowing how frequently I'll have to stop to check for the pink of my son's skin.

The nurse on the other line of the phone that day simply hangs up after directing me to a breastfeeding support group.

I have a number of follow-ups with my doctors, but I am never once screened for any type of postpartum mental illness. This, despite the fact that I check all the boxes for high risk. History of infertility: *check*. Complicated pregnancy: *check*. Preterm delivery requiring an extended hospital stay: *check*. First-time mom: *check*. The anxiety that fills my body leaves little space for anything else. I have never experienced a madness like this, and it distorts my ability to self-diagnose.

THERE ARE FEW MOMENTS OF REPRIEVE. EVEN WITH MY SON strapped to my chest as we venture out on sunny winter days for short walks, an act I perform in an attempt at normalcy, I pause every couple of steps to feel for his chest rising against mine. I check to make sure his face is still a vibrant pink and not a dusky blue. If I cannot have my son in my arms, I can only rest if he is in Joey's care. Knowing he is under the watchful eye of the only other person who has witnessed our son cheat death lets me stumble off to bed for a few hours of unbroken sleep. This is often the only sleep I get each night, and the only thing that keeps me from succumbing to full-blown mania. Even with a baby in my arms, his cries and coos tangible proof that he is alive, I am not convinced my son is here to stay. I have been wrong too many times before. Positive pregnancy tests turned negative, heartbeats that slowed to a stop, water breaking too soon. My fear of death, his death, creeps in from all corners of whatever room we are in. I know how death can strike anyone, at any time.

I read story after story about children dying from Sudden Infant Death Syndrome (SIDS) during these hazy few months. I convince myself that Teddy will be next if I don't stay on alert. These are stories of mothers waking in the morning realizing their infant has not woken as usual, only to find them cold and blue when they go into their room. I picture the wails, the frantic call to 911, the CPR performed all the way to the hospital. I hear the sound of ribs cracking and I hold my breath while a paramedic attempts to secure an airway. I hear the mothers' unnatural screams when they are told by a solemn doctor that nothing more can be done. I picture impossibly small white coffins buried under willow trees and a stone monument that becomes part of family legacy. It is dark and disturbing to spend so much time thinking about my son's death, but it is comforting to prepare for the worst. From the very first days of my pregnancy, I was so sure my child would never be born, and any day with him alive feels like borrowed time.

The one silver lining in all of this, even as it fills me with dread, is that my anxiety gives me an overwhelming appreciation for each moment. I am grateful to be woken at two and three and then again at four in the morning by a screaming infant because it means I have a screaming infant. I carry him in my arms everywhere I go because I have a baby to carry. I marvel at his growth in those early days. When he graduates from wearing the impossibly small preemie clothes to the newborn baby clothes I bought months before, I whisper, *Grow, baby, grow!*, so proud that he is gaining weight. I feel as though my whole job, the reason for my being, is to keep my son alive. And I don't realize that I am barely surviving it.

My first panic attack happens a month after we bring Teddy home from the hospital. I have spent the four previous weeks adjusting to life as a mom at home, undergoing a hibernation of sorts. I carried him everywhere, mimicking what would have been happening had he not been born prematurely, and I have no desire to leave the house.

We decide to take Teddy on his first adventure, to a friend's birthday brunch. We imagine it will be a good opportunity to show off our beautiful baby, who is no longer tethered to IV pumps and monitors. I bundle Teddy in his warmest outfit and sit beside him in the back seat while Joey drives us to the restaurant, like we're in a taxi.

When we arrive, Teddy is sound asleep, as most newborns are during the day, and we pull a warm cover over his car seat to protect his face from the wind. We run quickly across the road to get inside. When we are in the doorway, I immediately pull off the cover to peek at my son.

His face is purple, his chest still.

Panic courses through me. "Joe, something's wrong!" I say. Joey glances at Teddy, who is still in his car seat, and then back at me, shrugging his shoulders in confusion. I stifle the urge to scream and I replay the lessons I learned in NICU, reminding myself that premature babies sometimes require stimulation to breathe again. I pull at the straps of the car seat frantically, cursing under my breath at my husband, who remains incompetent beside me. I feel the straps resist against my panic, but finally they loosen, and I unclick the buckle holding them in place. I will lay my son on the ground to perform CPR while someone calls 911.

When I finally pull Teddy free, he stretches his arms upward and yawns contentedly, readjusting himself with his hands behind his head and smacking his lips. He settles into my arms and remains asleep, his chest rising with ease. His skin pink, full of life.

I hold onto Teddy the entire time we eat brunch, clinging to him fiercely in my right arm and feeding myself in tiny bites with my left hand. I force myself to smile and nod my head when someone is speaking near me. My heart is racing the entire time and I long to be back in our home where I can properly assess my baby for brain damage and evaluate why he stopped breathing. I remember wishing my friend a happy birthday, but beyond that I cannot tell you what I ate or how long we spent at the table. I am panicked the entire time, focused on calming my breathing and counting my baby's breaths in a restaurant that feels too loud and too bright.

Once Joey and I return home with Teddy still sleeping, I pace in our living room. I cry, circling the coffee table like a caged lion. Joey keeps trying to tell me to calm down, and I roar, "Something is really wrong!" I begin to dress Teddy in his warm clothes again, and I tell Joey we are heading to the hospital.

"But Jo, he's fine." Joey gestures to our contented baby who is now awake because I have dressed him, and his legs kick playfully as he coos.

"Start the car," I demand, staring icily at my husband. He looks like he isn't sure who I am, but he goes outside to scrape off the windshield, which has already frozen over in the brief time we have been home.

Once Joey is outside, I pace the living room once again. I look at my son, counting his breaths, and wonder, for the first time, if it is possible that I have imagined it all.

But he looked so blue, I think, *and he wasn't breathing. I know he wasn't.* I shake my head, wondering how my brain could have created a scene that had never existed.

When Joey returns, holding my coat in his hand, I am sitting on the couch and I have unbundled Teddy, who is back to sleep. I am chewing my nails, my knees drawn to my chest, and I don't look up when Joey sits beside me.

"Aren't we going?" he asks, with more kindness than I deserve.

"I think you're right," I reply quietly, still not making eye contact. "He's fine. Maybe nothing even happened."

I put my head in my hands. I have always been such a rational person, a woman who has studied and believes in science. I have always felt grounded, my feet firmly planted in reality with my thoughts and feelings rooted in what is tangible, what is real. This feels wildly irrational. Joey puts his arm around me to give me a hug before heading back outside to turn off the car.

After our brief restaurant outing, I barely leave the house for the remainder of the winter. I become a recluse, managing our daily lives from the comfort of my home by ordering groceries online and inviting friends to visit me in my living room. It takes several months for the adrenaline from that day in the restaurant to stop coursing through my body, and even though I manage to find a way to cope as the months go on, I am never quite the same.

I CONTINUE TO SEE HEATHER ONCE A WEEK, AND SHE TEACHES me to write during the moments I feel overwhelmed by worry. She tells me to make lists of what I am feeling, of what I can control and what I cannot. She says that naming my fears might allow me to regain a sense of balance in my life. She compares my anxiety to having vertigo.

"When someone has vertigo, their inner mechanism for feeling steady is broken. When the world is suddenly tumbling around them, they can't close their eyes to regain their balance. That will only make it worse. They need to try and look at a focal point, to focus on things beyond themselves. Your anxiety is like that. Your brain is telling you things that aren't true, so you can't turn inward. By stating things out loud, or writing them down, you are forced to re-evaluate what is real and what is not. It might help give you some balance when you are feeling overly worried."

I make lists in my journal when I am overcome with the fear that Teddy will stop breathing again, that he isn't growing or developing, that he could be gravely sick or in trouble. I rattle off the truths of a moment, repeating them in my head until I feel my heart rate slow and my world beginning to steady.

He is safe right now.
He is growing.
I have no control over the inner workings of his body.
If anything happens, I will handle it.
I have handled hard things before.
I am a good mom.

Teddy has recently started to ask me, "Are you okay?" It sounds innocent and sweet coming from his mouth, but only I know it is the echo of my anxiety. A parroting of the question I ask him regularly. When he's too quiet in his car seat. When he's wandered into the other room and I hear his feet stumble beneath him. When he crawls into my lap unprompted, laying his head on my shoulder.

Are you okay? Are you okay? Are you okay?

My need to hear him say "I'm okay, Mama" is my anxiety untethered. There will come a day when I won't always know the answer. My son will grow up and he will go places, he will make friends, sneak a sip of beer, travel, hopefully fall in love. I won't always be there to know if he's all right, and I need to be okay with that. I am learning to reign in my fear, to realize that my love for him does not need to be entwined with my fear of losing him.

17

▼

"I'M NOT ALWAYS DWELLING ON THE BAD," I TELL HEATHER during one of our weekly appointments. I have just finished telling her about the morning I had with Teddy. He was sweet and loving, and I shirked every other responsibility for hours, reading him stories, playing endless games of chase, letting the house get messy with our play. I felt nothing but joy all morning. I've being seeing Heather for months and I don't want to only speak of the sadness in my life anymore.

"Sometimes," I continue, "all I can think of is how happy I am to have him. I am overwhelmed by it." I pause to take a sip of my still-warm coffee, considering how I can best describe what it is I am feeling.

"It's like I'm split into two people. One is deeply sad about what I've gone through, and the other is incredibly happy to have my son. We're the same person, obviously, but sometimes I feel like a totally different person one hour to the next. I don't know if that makes any sense."

Heather props her elbow on the armrest of her chair and places her chin in her hand. She covers her mouth partially, her fingers stroking her bottom lip as though she is deep in thought. When she does this, I am reminded of a university professor I once had who, before making a point, would clear his throat and stroke his lip for what felt like minutes. I always felt it was pretentious, a way for him to make a display of his own intelligence, a grandiose flexing of his academic muscles, but in this office, I am thinking none of these things. Heather has my full attention. Her words are always insightful. They are worth waiting for.

"Think of your life as a tapestry, Joanne. Picture every life event you go through and every experience you have as a colour. When you're grieving after your miscarriages, your tapestry turns all one colour. Your life is overcome with that one thing. As time goes on, you're able to weave in more colours, like the morning you just described with Teddy."

I envision the tapestry that Heather described. I picture the weeks following a miscarriage as a dark blue, nearly black, thread that creates a void, almost an absence of colour. When I think of the morning with my son, I see a bright yellow being woven in between the stretches of dark. Each colour is distinct and yet they are connected together seamlessly, the tapestry of my life filled with times of intense sadness and immeasurable joy.

TIME PASSES IN A WAY IT NEVER HAS BEFORE. IT IS MEASURED against my son, who is constantly changing, growing. Each season passing is no longer a marker of my life but of my son's, of my life as his mother. It is not time that has changed, it is me. My days are now bound by nap times and diaper changes, playtime and snacks. They feel endless, and yet the moment the sun slips below the horizon each day I am left wondering where the hours have gone. There are times I look at him and already miss who he is now. It's like watching a flower unfold. He is becoming more of who he is with every passing day, and I feel as though I am meeting him, new, each morning.

The nights when I woke hourly to nurse a wrinkly newborn are now gone, fading more with each day. I get only glimpses of Teddy's newborn self now, mostly when he is sleeping, the way his hands clasp behind his head, and when he rolls onto his belly, landing in the most perfect child's pose; it's as though I can see him at every age in those moments. The way he arches his back, lifting his arms in a deep stretch after napping in his car seat, I can see the premature baby being lifted from the incubator, performing the same sleepy ritual.

When Teddy is nearly six months old, the weather is finally warm enough for Joey and I to take our son outside for a first we never knew was a part of parenthood: Teddy's first real experience of nature, the feeling of earth and grass against bare feet. We step into our front yard, listening to the wind rustle the leaves in the trees, and watch as a fat bumblebee bounces along the peonies in the garden. When I lower Teddy onto the grass, Joey films the moment with anticipation and we watch with excitement as the soles of our son's feet hit the tiny blades of grass. His feet instantly recoil at the tickle and he tucks his legs in. My own toes curl in response, as though we are still sharing one body.

Teddy first tastes lemon when he is eight months old. I watch him grab the lemon slice I place on his high chair, using a pudgy fist to thrust the sour fruit into his mouth with a newfound coordination. When he wrinkles his nose and grimaces, I feel my own mouth salivate in response. He peers at the fruit in his hand, the juices seeping from between his clenched fingers, and brings the lemon to his mouth again. He laughs, his tiny fists banging the plastic tray, delighted by the potency of the flavour. He still loves the taste of citrus, sneaking sips of lemon juice when he's helping me make supper.

I watch Teddy's growth with a mixture of amazement, sadness, and a pride incomparable to anything I have ever felt for myself. The moment I first hear him say "Mama," which comes out as "A-ma," tears spill from the corners of my eyes. He has finally found the word for who I am, who I will always be.

His life has become so entwined with my own, yet I can already feel the slow separation as we hurtle toward school years, adolescence, and the moment he leaves the home we have built for him. I feel that I am made for motherhood in a way that you step into a pair of jeans and you know they fit just right. Motherhood, for me, is not the ultimate sacrifice of my body or my time: those things I happily give to my son. The sacrifice will be in letting him go. I long to hold, cradle, and protect him for life, but to love him is to allow him to find his own place in the world without me. Like the babies I lost, I will one day have to let go of my living son as well. It is a heartache that every mother must endure, and it is only the strength of motherly love that makes it bearable.

One night, when Teddy is two, he is overtired, and nothing will settle him at bedtime. I try holding him, but he squirms and is uncomfortable in my arms. I put him into his crib, laying on the floor beside it, but he stands and cries while looking at me on the floor. I try rubbing his back and singing to him, but nothing seems to work. I step into the crib to lie on the small mattress beside him, hoping my body will provide some comfort. In this position, his body relaxes, and his cries turn to sniffles. He pulls my arm across his body, wrapping himself in a hug, but pushes my face further away. I move to get out of his crib, thinking he doesn't want me there anymore, but as I start to get up, he tugs on my arm saying, "Just go, don't go, Mama." I couldn't have said it better myself.

I AM IMMENSELY PROUD TO BE MY SON'S MOTHER. I AM PROUD of things for which I can take no credit, like the way his hair curls into perfect ringlets and how he scrunches his nose when he smiles. Teddy is an agreeable child. Mild-tempered and like-able, always contemplating a situation and waiting before he tries anything new. One day we attend a play group at the local library, filled with children of various ages. The teacher is animated, playing music and dancing while we enter the brightly lit room. Most children sit on the rainbow mat at front of the room, the parents filling the chairs behind them. Teddy has no interest in sitting on the mat. He sits beside me instead, his back straight. He is interested, I can tell, but also trepidatious.

The class begins with a dance party. The teacher puts on the "Hokey Pokey" and the kids on the mat are twirling, jumping, and freezing while making silly faces at each other. I clap and sing along, sneaking a glance at Teddy, who is watching intensely. I tickle him slightly, trying to get him to dance with me in his seat. As a child, I would have been the girl in the front row, the first one to join in and do what the teacher asked. This moment is a powerful reminder that Teddy is his own person and not an extension of myself.

Toward the end of the class, the teacher passes out small egg-shaped shakers to all the kids from a bin held in his arms. Teddy waits until the crowd of children dissipates, then slips out of his chair and walks to the front of the room, quietly taking two shakers from the bin. He returns to his chair and he hands me the yellow one, keeping the blue one for himself, saying, "Here you go, Mama."

"Thanks, buddy." I smile, touched by his thoughtfulness.

The kids in the class are shaking their eggs wildly, some are tossing them into the air and watching as they crash noisily to the floor. I enthusiastically shake mine, trying to demonstrate how much fun this is to my serious boy. Teddy shakes his slowly, getting a feel for engaging in the group.

By the end of the class, Teddy has slipped out of the chair beside me and is sitting among the other kids. They are listening to a story about monkeys going to space. He turns back to look at me, a small smile on his lips. I make a motion with my hands that is a cross between a prayer and a silent clap, feeling so proud of him for joining at his own pace.

When the class is over, he helps the other kids put the toys into the brightly coloured storage bins and then quietly thanks the teacher. He reaches for my hand and we walk out of the library together. He is teaching me how there are so many different ways of being. That we all have our place.

I am learning to walk through the world in a pace that mimics my toddler's. We admire cracks on the sidewalk where dandelions push through. We discover cobwebs with dewdrops that look like bubbles. Moths are white butterflies. Bumblebees are friends to be cared for. Our garden is full of surprises and things to learn. Pine trees are prickly, and slugs are slippery when you place them in the palm of your hand. Buttercups and daises aren't weeds; they are gathered in a pudgy fist and handed to me as a beautiful floral arrangement. I place them in a jar filled with tap water and they earn the coveted spot in the middle of our table. Teddy smiles with pride when he sees how happy they make me, how grateful I am.

Teddy doesn't like being messy. I take him to an art class one month to teach him that getting our hands dirty can be fun. I encourage him to do so during the class by dipping his fingers into the bright colours of the paint, but his favourite part is when the teacher hands us a rag and his hands get wiped clean. I am still learning to pay attention to who he is.

He takes his first steps at eleven months old. As soon as he can stand, he grabs hold of our hands, using us for stability as he paces around our house. He has been determined to walk for weeks. When he takes his first unsteady steps, his arms raised above his head for balance and his legs moving in a shaky gait, Joey and I clap and cheer for our brave toddler.

I take Teddy to a baby gymnastics class, and he clings to me the entire time. The other toddlers go into the arms of their delightful teacher, Hannah, who is funny and sweet with each of them. Teddy cannot be convinced to go to her outstretched arms. I have learned not to push him, that he will do it in his own time. One month into classes, he toddles over to Hannah when she puts her arms out to him, and she smiles with the satisfaction that he has finally trusted her. She smiles wildly at me, Teddy in her arms, and I clap my hands in encouragement.

He is curious and quizzical about the world around him, wanting to know what things are made of and how the world works. His wonder at learning new things delights me.

When baking together, I let Teddy lick the spoon, feeling slightly fearful of the raw egg, but I ignore my worry and pass him the spoon anyway. He grins, licking it greedily. He is my steadfast companion in the early years of his life. We spend more time together than with anyone else. He is learning how to crack an egg, the shells landing amid the butter and sugar before I scoop them out with my fingers. Teddy points to my dirtied fingers and with a wrinkled nose he says, "Mama, look." He still doesn't like getting his hands messy. I keep a wet cloth on the island of our kitchen so he can easily wipe his hands when they become sticky with batter.

I open the oven door, using my one hand to slide the muffin tray onto the wire rack while I stretch the other out behind me. A protective stance in case Teddy should disobey my warnings about the hot oven. With the door closed, I set the timer.

He stands on a stool over the sink as we clean up together, letting the warm water pool into a small bowl which he dumps repeatedly over the dirty utensils. He loves the water. To pass the time on days that feel long, I let him play in the sink for an hour, mopping up the water that inevitably pools on the floor beneath him.

The timer dings loudly and I pull the muffins from the oven, setting them on a rack on the counter. I break one open to make it cool faster, as Teddy always wants to eat them right away. When it has cooled down enough, he takes a bite, sinking his teeth into the soft top. He smiles with a mouthful of muffin and says, "So good, Mama." He doesn't care that the mix came from a box or that in ten minutes they will harden up because I always over-mix muffin batter. He is delighted that we made something together. He finds such joy in things so small, and I find joy in him.

18

▼

WE TAKE TEDDY TO ALBERTA A MONTH BEFORE HE TURNS TWO.
We want to visit the friends we've kept in touch with, most of
whom have children of their own, and introduce Teddy to the
fresh mountain air we breathed in during our twenties. After
landing in Edmonton, we drive to the Rockies with our group
of friends to take the five kids on a hike. We laugh at how cute
they look in their snowsuits, how difficult it is for them to move
with their arms and legs splayed out like starfish. I take a photo
next to Kellie, our toddlers strapped to our backs, with her older
daughter grinning for the camera in front of us.

After more than an hour on the trail, we have barely moved.
Mittens keep falling off small hands or toddlers stumble, needing snow brushed off their rosy cheeks. Boots fall off and need
to be put back on socked feet that are now cold and wet. By
this time, three of the children are crying, including Teddy, and
Joey suggests it might be time to turn back. The hike will have
to wait. Back at the hotel, we all pile into a hot tub with a view
of the mountains and the kids calm down. Water has a way of
turning bad moods good and crying toddlers into giggling ones.
It is snowing as we sit in the warm, bubbling water, the air thick
with steam. Winter comes early in the Rockies, and Teddy looks
with wonder as the early November snow makes everything
around us sparkle.

We drive back to the city, showing Teddy our favourite sights
around Edmonton, telling him how Mama and Dada spent years
of their life in a city that vaguely felt like home. We drive past
our old apartment and picture our younger selves tucked inside,

living together for the first time, playing house. We take Teddy to an amusement park inside a mall and sit him atop a plastic horse. We put a dollar into the slot, and as soon as the horse lurches to life, Teddy cries and puts up his arms, saying, "Off, off." He watches the horse move from the safety of my arms, and once it goes still, he climbs back on. His insistence to enjoy the ride motionless makes us laugh. We relax while staying with our friends in their home, watching as Teddy plays with their young daughters, fitting in seamlessly as children do. And I imagine him playing with his own siblings someday.

When Teddy was still an infant, Joey and I spoke about having more children with the certainty we believed it was.

"I think we should have three," I said, holding a sleeping Teddy against my chest. Teddy's age was still being measured in weeks and our house acted like an incubator while we spent the winter tucked safely inside. Joey smiled on the couch beside us, placing his hand on Teddy's head.

"Let's start with two and go from there."

We don't mention how hard it was to have Teddy, how our first two losses and our son's premature arrival should not be dismissed so casually. We were drunk with love for our son and we magically believed my body had been repaired by bearing our child. That Teddy's birth had somehow paved the way for more children to survive, opened up the possibility of others. We believed that lightning could strike twice. In my postpartum appointments, my doctor reinforced our beliefs by telling us how likely it was that we would have a second child now that we had one. She told us what we wanted to hear, handing us the hope for a future as though she were God. We loved our son with a fervour that made us hungry to experience this again. We were greedy for more.

Joey grew up imagining his life as the father of more than one child. We both hold the same image of our family in our minds, a shared dream that we began building during our first date years ago. By having Teddy, our dream feels even more like a certainty than ever before.

We both know we'd be happy for our children to be close in age—Joey is two years younger than his brother, and my three siblings and I are spaced out evenly as well. We reflect on our plans to adopt, and realize that truly, they were a way for me to survive those childless months, but not what we actually want. Our adoption paperwork begins collecting dust on a shelf and we never pick it up again. We long for a baby who might look like Teddy, a second child made from our love. We naively believe that since we had done it once before, we can do it again.

Before leaving for our trip to Edmonton, I buy the same ovulation tests I used before having Teddy. I begin tracking my cycle, certain that things will be different this time.

ON OUR FOURTH DAY IN ALBERTA, I TAKE ONE OF THE ovulation tests. The smiley face tells me I am ovulating. Joey and I make love amid the mountains. Afterwards, we smile at each other, saying how great it would be if our second baby were connected to our second home. We fly home from our vacation, and even with the hope for another baby filling my thoughts, I am surprised when my period fails to arrive weeks later. It feels too good to be true.

It is late November, when the day's light disappears long before supper, and with my hands shaking in the dim evening light, I tear open the package of a pregnancy test.

Positive.

Knowing Joey is about to arrive home, I grab a scrap piece of paper and scrawl a few words in crayon and fold the note in half. I hear the front door open and Teddy say "Dada!"

Joey walks in the door and I hand Teddy the piece of paper, whispering, "Give this to Dada." I can barely stand still in anticipation. Teddy hands Joey a note that reads, *Dada, I'm going to be a big brother!* Joey looks at me and I hold the positive pregnancy test in the air like a conductor waiting to begin a symphony. Joey lifts me off the ground in an excited hug, swinging me around like he did on our wedding day. Teddy, always ready for excitement, jumps around our legs with his hands in the air, saying, "Me too! Me too!" We scoop him into our arms, embracing our soon-to-be family of four.

That night, I tiptoe out of Teddy's room after he falls asleep and join Joey on the couch. We speak about the baby, but the certainty we felt hours earlier is starting to crack beneath the weight of our fears. At one point, Joey puts his hand on my stomach and says, "I will love you so much if you are ever born."

If.

We use words to protect us from what we fear most. We speak in sentences that imply hope but are tainted with fear. We act as though words can dull the pain of losing a baby that is already born in our minds. When we go to bed, I turn toward Joey and ask if we can spend the few minutes before we fall asleep speaking as though this baby is a sure thing. I want to drop the language that is intended to protect us and allow the last moments of the day to be happy thoughts of our family of four. And so, we speak about names we like and the age gap between our two children. We discuss when and how we will tell Teddy about his younger brother or sister. We think ahead to how we'll have a newborn on our family vacation the following summer and consider booking bigger accommodations to house our growing family. We fall asleep happy, thinking about how fiercely we loved Teddy the moment he was born, certain we'll feel that love again.

A few days later I am filling treat bags for Teddy's second birthday party. It is *Sesame Street*–themed, so I've ordered a large Elmo balloon that will dance around our home for the next few weeks. On the Saturday of his party, the icing I use for the cupcakes will stain our lips a deep blue, reminding me of the swim classes my parents made me take as a child.

When I was five, we moved to a lakefront house where I spent much of my childhood. Adamant we wouldn't drown, my parents made me and my two older siblings take swimming lessons in a lake. My mom drove us to our lessons in the early hours of the morning, where we'd wade into the frigid waters of June. We learned how to navigate unexpected drop-offs and slippery rocks, and how to manage the leeches that clung to our bare ankles in the ice-cold water. We swam until our lips turned blue, our teeth chattering in our skulls like ventriloquist dummies'.

My mom would stand on the edge of the lake with blankets and towels, waiting for us to run toward her when our class was over. It was my favourite part. I ran without feeling in my legs toward my smiling mom, her arms outstretched, waiting. When she wrapped a towel around me tightly, her hands rubbing my shoulders through the soft fabric, a warmth enveloped me, making the lessons bearable. I could tolerate the cold because she was at the water's edge, waiting. Her warm embrace my reward. It would take hours for my lips to return to their natural colour, long after I changed into warm clothes and drank the hot chocolate my mom kept in a bright red Thermos. I would look in the mirror at the darkened hue of my mouth, running my fingertips along my bottom lip, trying to wipe the colour away.

In our dining room now, I create a treat-bag assembly line. Well-organized piles of plastic dinosaurs, stickers, and bubbles are spread across the table. I reach for a purple triceratops to place into one of bags with a smiling Big Bird on the front when I bend over in pain. The bag drops to the floor. A vise has wrapped itself around my middle and is squeezing me tightly. I undo the button on my jeans, trying to find some relief. I feel the pain retreat slowly, like a wave receding, and a trickle of fluid hits my underwear.

I call Joey at work while sitting on the toilet, my head in my hands.

"I'm bleeding," I say flatly, looking down at my underwear stained a bright red.

He sighs into the phone. "I'm so sorry."

Joey drives home and Teddy, who has just woken up from his nap, is excited to see him. We turn on the TV and cheerful nursery rhymes fill the air while Joey and I sit silently on the couch. The high-pitched hiss of the kettle sounds, and Joey goes to the kitchen. Minutes later he returns, handing me a hot cup of tea that I take in both hands. I am shivering even though our house is warm. I sip my tea, trying to stop the sadness from taking me in its grip.

I recognize my grief and it taints everything black. The next morning is as dark as night, but I'm sure that can't be right. Memory is fallible, unreliable at the best of times, and even more when you are overcome with grief. The darkness is familiar, as though a houseguest who always trashes my home has come to stay. *At least I know what to expect*, I think, as I try to make myself believe this miscarriage will be easier than the last. As if I can swiftly hide all the breakables in my home to prevent them from being smashed by my violent guest.

I MAKE AN APPOINTMENT WITH DR. STEWART, WHO CARED FOR Teddy as an infant, and I keep my head down in the waiting room. I answer her questions robotically, feeling disconnected from the words I am saying out loud.

"Yes, I'm sure this is another miscarriage."

"Yes, I'm sure I am pregnant."

After performing a physical, Dr. Stewart starts to offer words of sympathy, but I cut her off, waving my hands, shooing her words away like mosquitoes.

"It's okay," I say. "Really."

I look away from her kind gaze to the dozens of baby photos taped to the wall. A shrine to all the babies she's helped deliver. As I leave her office for an urgent ultrasound, she tells me to take care. I don't respond except to close the door quietly behind me, putting space between myself and the babies who survived.

During the ultrasound, I am unable to feel anything except the cold speculum and the probe as it pokes around inside me. The exam lasts only minutes and I don't need to hear what the doctor has to say. I know my baby is gone.

When I return home, Joey meets me in the front hall, looking at me expectantly. He has a dishtowel over his shoulder and his sleeves rolled up. I can smell the pasta he is cooking, a favourite meal his grandmother used to make, and even its smell is comforting. I shake my head in response to his silent question, unable to stop my tears from falling. He wraps his arms around me, like my mom after swim class, and I bury my head deep into his chest. I pull away a few moments later and I can see I've left a mascara stain on his white T-shirt. I try wiping it away, but it's no use. Joey goes into the kitchen to finish making supper, and I sit down beside Teddy as he plays with his cars on the living room floor. I hug him tightly, breathing in the scent of his head, telling myself I can't feel sad because I have him.

With Teddy asleep that night, I crawl under the covers of my bed and I feel the enormity of what I have lost. The bed shakes with my sadness. I no longer find comfort in the familiarity of pain; it feels like I will never find relief from its searing ache. I clutch my stomach and it is tense, the physical pain reminding me that my body still has to purge whatever is left inside. I hear Joey flick on the bathroom light, and then water flowing from the faucet as he brushes his teeth. He crawls into bed beside me and wraps his arms around my body, a body that is failing us both, his hands overlapping mine.

I wake the next morning with Joey's arms still around me and tears dried on my face. I hear Teddy stirring in his crib, and I rise to perform the role of a woman who is not grieving the loss of her unborn child. I make coffee and breakfast, playing music loudly from our record player to drown out my thoughts. I dance with Teddy in the living room, feeling like an actor in a play, except I have never been very good at acting. My one success came in sixth grade when my teacher, Mrs. Turner, chose me to star as Lady Macbeth in our end-of-year production. My acting career ended at curtain call. I have never been able to convincingly be anything other than myself.

I do laundry, letting Teddy sit in the middle of the basket, and throw the freshly folded clothes onto the floor. I pick them up, folding them again and again, enjoying how happy this makes him. I reach over and hug him, feeling my eyes sting, and he hugs me back tightly, perhaps feeling my sadness. When I lay him down for his afternoon nap, I retreat to the bathroom to cry.

The following day, I return to work. I take more Advil than is recommended and a few kind co-workers stop me in the hallway, asking if I am all right.

"I'm fine," I say through pursed lips. I try smiling, but the dark circles under my eyes and the pallor of my skin give me away. When I tell them what happened, I shake my head when they suggest I go home.

I take Maddy for a walk after work. I can't stop thinking about a story I recently read, by a mother who tragically lost her toddler son who had been born prematurely. As she tells it, one day, months after her son died, she was walking to her car when she came across a large, white feather. She was struck by the feather and bent over to pick it up. Once inside her car, she googled what finding a feather meant, and the first search item said, "When feathers appear, angels are near." How beautiful, the woman mused in her essay, and she described feeling close to her son in that moment.

Maddy and I continue walking along a path in the woods near our home. Parts of the ground are newly frozen, causing me to look down to help navigate the slippery path. As I step forward, I notice a small white feather near my foot. I stop abruptly, making Maddy lurch on the leash. I smile, thinking maybe it is a sign from the embryo I've just lost. I bend to pick it up, but I notice the red glistening on its tip. Looking further ahead in the woods, I can see more feathers littering the ground, as though someone has just had a pillow fight. Suddenly the scene comes into focus and I take in the sight of the obliterated carcass of a small bird.

Maddy is pulling, trying to get closer to the decomposing body, and I struggle to pull her away on the icy ground. Once we are several feet from the dead bird, I start to cry. What I have found on the path represents all of the ugliness of my miscarriages. The experiences I had, the grief I feel over my lost pregnancies, these are much more represented by a pulverized, half-eaten, dead bird than by a single, beautiful feather.

I return home, hearing Teddy and Joey playing in the bath upstairs, and I wonder if I will ever feel normal again.

"PEOPLE WITH ONLY ONE CHILD ARE AMATEURS," A STRANGER tells me one day soon after, smiling as if I am in on the joke.

I am eating lunch with a good friend, Erin. Erin has turned around in her chair to speak with a friend of hers who walked by our table, and I'm sipping my coffee when I make eye contact with the woman who is sitting at the table beside us. The restaurant is small, so there is very little space between us. I am still bleeding heavily, racing to and from the bathroom to change my pads and stifle sobs, all while my body ejects pieces of my wanted baby. I apologize with every flush of the toilet, heartbroken to leave them behind in a public washroom. I am emotionally raw and sitting with one of my safest friends. Erin has never been afraid to follow me into the dark to make sure I'm not alone. She is always willing to climb into that hole with me, and she's been a constant source of comfort since I lost the first of my babies.

On our way to lunch, we dodge into bathrooms while walking down the busy street and Erin gives me the time I need to manage the physical side effects of my miscarriage, the miscarriage I am still having. We wander into bookstores and she recommends a book on grief that I read that night, filled with a sense of being seen. She allows me to steer every conversation back to my miscarriage. She takes such care of the emotional side of my loss and she gives me space to breathe, a laugh that fills my bones with relief. She offers me the belief that I am not alone.

We have just ordered lunch when the woman on the bench beside me overhears a comment I make about my son and asks me how many children I have. After telling her, "Just the one!" she passes judgment that I don't have more. I feel less-than—an amateur—as though I am not a real mom. I know she does not, cannot, know the hurt that her words inflict. We are all assumed to be fertile until we produce no offspring by a certain age. And any non-parents are presumed to be either infertile or selfish, perhaps one and the same. Women of child-bearing age have to bear so much judgment from friends and strangers alike.

When are you going to have children?
You're not getting any younger.
Miscarriages are even more common as you get older.
You're going to want to give that boy a sibling before he gets too used to being an only child.

Women are told in so many ways that we are meant to procreate, to have more than one child—but not *too* many—and to have them spaced out within an acceptable length of time. We see this narrative play out on television, in movies, in books—everywhere, all the time. After I tell someone my son has recently turned two, they look at my abdomen expectantly and say, "It won't be long till you have your second!"

I am no longer childless, but I still long for the babies I lost, the ones I still wish for. I am a grieving mother, but I am also a mother with a child on her hip. My arms know the loneliness of being empty, and yet they are filled with the little boy who calls me Mama. I am an enigma, someone even I am not familiar with. I have never met another woman like me, and the isolation of it forces me to retreat inwards for several months. I hide behind smiles and polite declines to social events. I learn how to say no, without needing to explain further. I am bereft after my third miscarriage, but I feel like I am not supposed to grieve because I have my son. I keep myself tucked away, trying to force the anger and sadness out, but it's like trying to stop the tide from coming. It always comes.

I feel like I have barely made it to motherhood, my body cooperating just long enough to allow me to have this life-altering experience. I am not a "regular" mom. I long to have a birth story that doesn't make people gasp. I don't fit in with the mothers who lament sibling rivalries or conflicting schedules or unplanned children. And I don't fit in with my friends who are childless by choice or by infertility. I oscillate between both being and not being a mom at regular intervals. With every pregnancy I am a new mother, and with every miscarriage I am, once again, without child. On the outside, I look like any other woman, but I'm not as intact as I once thought. I am not quite who I appear to be.

Oh, you have a bicornuate uterus, a new ultrasound tech will say when she sees the unusual contour of my womb on the screen.

You've had surgery, doctors announce when they see the scars littered across my abdomen like stars in the night sky.

As a toddler, I had surgery to remove a benign tumour from my ear. Any time a new doctor looked in my ear they'd say, "Oh wow, what happened in here?"

My body is adept at keeping secrets. Tumours hidden inside ears, a misshapen uterus, babies that die before they can be born.

As the days turn into weeks, I give myself permission to cry, to sit still, to scream when I am alone in the car. I do everything to try and move forward except giving myself the time to properly grieve. Joey and I speak passionately about the future again, about the second child we long for, the second child we will have. We allow ourselves to reminisce about the baby we just lost, but we focus on the life we want. The one with our son, his future sibling, and each other. It will be a good life, a great life in fact, and we hold onto hope despite our most recent loss. It is hope, and the desire to avoid the searing pain of grief, that drives us to try and get pregnant again only weeks after my miscarriage. It is hope that wraps itself around my shoulders when I stand in my bathroom staring in disbelief at another positive pregnancy test. But it is fear that fills my throat.

It is one month after our third miscarriage. I look in the mirror at my frightened reflection, preparing to tell Joey about the new baby I am so afraid will never be born. Before I go downstairs, where he is waiting for me to tell him what our future might hold, I allow myself a moment to consider, *What if this one makes it?*

19

▼

I DREAM I AM IN A CAR ACCIDENT. MY CAR FLIPS AND AFTER it lands, I turn to look at the back seat, frantic. Teddy is fine, sitting in his car seat, smiling. I unclick my seat belt, open my car door, and quickly walk around the side of the car. I pull him from his seat, hugging him tightly, relieved he is all right. I hear a noise. I walk over to investigate, Teddy clinging to me like a koala cub. I look down and see a baby lying on the ground, crying, near the front wheel of our car. I gasp, reaching for the infant, who appears untouched. A screeching sound makes me stop. I look over my shoulder and see a car heading toward us. I race to the edge of the road with Teddy in my arms and I turn my back to protect him, burrowing my head into his shoulder, bracing for impact. I hear the crunch of metal as the cars collide behind us. The baby's cries stop.

I wake, trying to shake the dream from my mind, and I reach for the bottle of hormones on my side table. Dr. Stewart's name is in the corner; they were prescribed days after my positive pregnancy test. I look outside at the frosty February morning and place my hand on my abdomen, thinking about the small life inside. I hear Teddy's cries from his crib. Joey rolls over and asks sleepily, "Is it my turn?"

"No, it's mine," I say softly, giving him a kiss on the cheek.

I am taking Teddy to the museum this morning. It has been cold all week and I want to get out of the house. When it's time to leave, I zip up his red, down-filled jacket, lifting his chin to close the zipper at the top, and pull his hat tightly over his ears. He grins.

The ground is frosty, slick, and Teddy doesn't like how his feet kept sliding beneath him. He stands with his arms in the air saying, "Mama, carry." His inability to pronounce his Rs gives him a Bostonian accent. It always makes me smile.

I heave him up, his weight heavy with all of his winter gear, and I start up the steps leading to our car. At the top, I lose my footing. A patch of ice beneath a fresh skiff of snow takes my legs from under me. I make a split-second decision: I pull Teddy toward my body tightly, rendering myself helpless. His body slams against mine as we land hard on the frozen ground, my body acting as a cushion for his. Teddy starts crying.

"Are you okay?" I ask, standing him on his feet, assessing him for any sign of injury. His lip is bleeding slightly, he bit it on impact, and I wipe it with my mitten. I breathe with relief when his cries stop and he becomes preoccupied with the snowflakes sticking to his blue wool mittens. The snow looks like tiny pieces of Styrofoam, as if someone has opened a package, the pieces filling the air and sticking to everything in sight.

I feel an ache in my hip and a sharp pain in my pelvis. I sit on the ice for a minute, trying to shake the feeling that something very bad has just happened.

Two days later, I start to bleed. Teddy and I are attending a parent-and-tot gymnastics class. I have been carrying around giant miscarriage pads, waiting for the moment to strike, but I have already bled through my pants by the time I escape to the bathroom with Teddy in my arms. He looks on with shock in his eyes and says "Uh-oh" when he sees the blood-filled toilet.

"It's okay, baby, it's okay," I whisper on repeat. I'm not sure which baby I am speaking to.

I grab our things and leave, deciding the big red mat, with its joyful soundtrack of babies and toddlers playing, is not the place to have a miscarriage. I drive home, my heart pounding, and though Teddy chats to me from his car seat the whole drive home, I don't hear a word he says. My ears are ringing as though a bomb has been detonated inside me. I pull into the driveway next to Joey's car and look inside it. Joey is sitting in the driver's seat, having forgotten his keys, locking himself out of the house.

Months earlier, we'd gone to a restaurant for supper and after returning home, realized we had both forgotten our keys. Teddy enjoyed our adventure around the perimeter of our house while we searched for the key we keep hidden outside. We used the spare key that night, forgetting to return it afterwards. Every couple of weeks, one of us would lock ourselves out of the house and we would be reminded, once again, that we needed to put it back. And we always forgot.

I step out of the car into the cold February air, unsure of what I am going to say. Joey gets out of his car, the door slamming behind him, and walks over to where I stand. He smiles at me sheepishly.

For a moment, I don't want to tell him. I know his smile will disappear, and that it will hurt him as deeply as it is hurting me. I can't keep anything from him, though, let alone this.

"I'm bleeding," I say.

The smile on his face disappears and his eyes fill with concern. "Oh, love…" he starts, but I cut him off.

"It's okay. I'm okay. I'm going to head to the hospital tonight, though. Do you think you can do bedtime?"

His face is still worried, but he nods his head and says, "Of course. Why don't we call your sister and I can go with you?"

I take Teddy out of his car seat and we slowly walk down the steps to the house, since he insists on walking on his own. The ever-independent toddler. He pauses and looks up at Joey, saying, "Dada home!" and we interrupt our conversation to smile and say, "You're right, Teddy. Dada's home!"

"No love, I can do this on my own. I got this." I say, smiling a bit too broadly, knowing Joey can see through it. He squeezes my hand in response.

I run upstairs and put on my miscarriage outfit of the season: comfortable black pants and an oversized black sweater. I throw my blood-stained jeans on the floor of the bathroom. When I return home later that night, I will place them in the sink filled with cold water. The laundry detergent will make the bathroom smell like a swimming pool. I will scrub my pants, sobbing, as I try to rid the fabric of its stains. I will watch the water in the sink turn brown from my own blood, and I'll leave them to soak overnight.

Before leaving for the hospital, I fill my bag with a water bottle, extra-large pads, and two books to keep my mind as occupied as possible. I come downstairs and Joey puts his arms around me.

"I'm going to do this one differently," I whisper in his ear. "I promise. I can do this one better."

I give Teddy a kiss and an extra-long hug and drive to the hospital alone. It is only then that I remember my dream from days earlier. The one where I saved the child in my arms, but I couldn't save the baby beyond my reach. The air is forced from my lungs in a sharp exhale and I put my hand flat against my chest as if I can blunt the pain of my heart breaking. I feel like that will always be my destiny: forever unable to save a baby from the car wreck of my body. But I had managed to pull my son free, hugging him tightly, keeping him safe.

In my dream, just before I woke, I walked away from the car wreck, singing softly into my son's curly hair. As I sang "Twinkle, Twinkle, Little Star," trying to calm myself just as much as my son, I wished desperately there was more I could have done for the baby we left behind.

I am in the waiting room of the ER when I am called to be seen in triage. I sit down on the chair next to the nurse's desk and she asks me perkily, "And what brings you in tonight?"

"I'm having a miscarriage," I say, looking at my hands.

She pauses her typing and looks at me. "Oh my," she says. "I'm so sorry." She asks me to explain how I know and how far along I am. I explain how this has happened three times before and that I am six and a half weeks pregnant. I tell her I am only here because I need to get the shot that does not seem to be helping preserve my pregnancies, otherwise I would have never stepped foot in this place.

When experiencing a miscarriage, my body sounds an alarm that I'm in the midst of a crisis. I can feel cramps, urges to push. It feels like I should be rushed in to be seen by a doctor immediately because my heart is pounding, and I feel desperate to hold onto the life inside. Since there is nothing that can stop a miscarriage from happening, I am told that what I am experiencing is not, in fact, urgent. It's as though I am forever being handed a yellow sheet from a nurse.

"Please take a seat in the waiting room, Mrs. Gallant."

There is nothing to do but wait.

When I see a doctor, I am told that my baby is still alive. I have a subchorionic hematoma, the same bruising I'd had with Teddy. I am sent home to do the only thing I am ever told to do. For three days, I hold onto the hope that this will become another baby, like my son. I return to the hospital a few days later and wait for the results. The nurse has brought me to a private room, and I am sitting awkwardly on the stretcher. I've left my winter coat on, feeling too vulnerable to take it off, and my foot is resting uncomfortably on the wheel below me. My arms are wrapped tightly around my body and I am bracing myself for what is to come. I am shivering through my warm layers.

The doctor walks in with a single sheet of paper in his hand. He sits on the chair in front of me, a move likely intended to comfort, but it makes me acutely aware that he is here to tell me bad news.

"Well," he starts, "your hormone levels have dropped to twenty-five hundred." He pauses, wondering whether I know what that means.

Days earlier, my hormone levels had been well above forty thousand, the message I was with child coursing through my body. As a veteran in the world of miscarriages, I do understand the gravity of what he is saying. A dramatic drop in hormone so early in a pregnancy can only mean one thing: the baby has died.

He looks at me with a furrowed brow, trying to determine whether I've understood the news he has carelessly tossed my way. My breathing is rapid and shallow, my panic-stricken face streaks with tears. I put my head in my hands, trying to absorb the shock, when the doctor stands and asks, "Does that sound good to you?" I imagine this is something he says routinely, though it is strikingly out of place in this context. Like when you accidentally say "Good, thanks" when someone simply says "Hello."

My crying stops for a second. I raise my head and I let out a tiny laugh at the absurdity of his question. He mumbles that obviously it probably isn't and something else I don't hear. I stand abruptly and he stops talking. My hands are shaking. My eyes narrow when I look at him, and his eyes dart away when I meet his gaze head on.

I hold up my hands to dismiss anything else he might have to say, and I announce, "I'm going to go now." He looks chastened while I walk out the double doors and out of that awful hospital room.

I gasp for breath in the bathroom across the hallway as I kneel on the filthy floor, clutching my soon-to-be-empty stomach. I stay like this for minutes, unable to stop my sobs. Knowing there is likely a line of people outside the door, I stand, put on my sunglasses, and walk out the door. I don't bother to hold it open for whoever goes in after. I somehow drive home, curl up in bed, and cry. I never feel more alone than in those first few hours after a life inside me has died.

IF MY HEART WAS CRACKED BEFORE THIS, MY FOURTH MISCAR-riage shatters it. It feels like those forgotten keys will never be replaced, forever locking me out of the family I long for. I become unrecognizable to Joey, and even to myself, and I struggle to get out of bed. I begin to believe that all of this is my fault. I hate my body, like I did when I was a child. Except instead of feeling ugly, I feel worthless. As if my inability to carry a pregnancy is a reflection of who I am as a person. I feel my confidence as a mother die as the last remains of my pregnancy leave my body. It is this fourth miscarriage that leads me to seek help from Heather, without being able to explain why this one feels so different from all the rest.

20

▼

"Do you often take responsibility for things that aren't your fault?" Heather asks me during our fifth therapy session together.

"No, not at all," I reply, without pause.

Heather stays silent, which, I have learned over the past month, means she either doesn't believe me or she thinks I am holding back. I look away from where she is seated in her grey armchair. It is tilted at a slight angle from where I sit, her crossed legs pointing at the door instead of directly at me. I imagine the arrangement of the room is meant to carefully encourage those sitting in my position to feel at ease. But I always feel nervous, regardless of how serene the room. I look over at the turquoise side table and a large clock tells me we have fifteen minutes left. I take a sip of my coffee and try to find comfort in the silence I know won't last.

"Let me put it another way," she tries again, being the first to break the silence. "Do you consider yourself to be responsible?"

"Yes…" I reply hesitantly, feeling like I am about to unwittingly make a confession.

"So, is it safe to say you put a lot of value on your ability to be a responsible person?"

I nod my response, still unsure what I am agreeing to.

"Okay. Now, consider the fact that being responsible is a trait that typically gets us places we want to go in life. If we are responsible by nature, we tend to do well in school, or at work, and in our personal relationships. It's good to have people rely on us. However, with every good trait we have, there is a dark counterpart. What can happen, without us even knowing, is that you may take responsibility for things when you shouldn't. Does that sound familiar to you?"

I nod in response and I nervously bite at my thumbnail. Heather is writing things down while I ruminate on what she is unveiling.

"I think," Heather says, interrupting my thoughts, "that the dark side of you being responsible is your need for control. You feel secure when you are in control and things are going well, but when you are in a situation that is uncontrollable, like your miscarriages, you blame yourself."

I am sobbing, unable to reply.

"You blame yourself for the loss of your babies, don't you?"

I nod and answer her in between sobs. "It's so much easier to blame myself than to accept I don't have control over any of this." I pause, grabbing a tissue before I can speak again. "I'm so scared that if my miscarriages aren't my fault, there isn't anything I can do to save them."

Heather lets me cry before she responds. "This isn't your fault, Joanne. I know you don't believe this right now, but it isn't. You have to accept that there is nothing you can do to save them."

When I get home, I write in my journal, *If I can't save them, it means nobody can. What does that mean for my hope? I am so sad.*

I end up on all fours in the shower that night, crying deep, guttural sobs, feeling pain with an intensity I have only ever imagined before.

In the days that follow, I turn to words for comfort. Ever since I was a child, I have been drawn to stories about loss and death. Reading them allowed me to embody other people's emotions briefly, fleetingly. I used other people's stories as a way to release whatever sadness I was carrying within me. A bully at school, a bad mark on a test, being the only girl cut from the field hockey team. They soothed me, even when I wasn't mourning, allowing me to feel less alone. I seek comfort from other people's stories like the way Teddy tucks his hands down the front of my shirt when he is sad or tired. His hands searching blindly for the solace my breasts once gave, my body giving him what my words and actions cannot.

When I was nine, my sister, Janet, and I spent hours watching figure skating on television. We spun around our living room, mimicking the athletes' movements, and we practiced our double axles in our shared bedroom, long after we were meant to be sleeping. One morning, in the midst of our figure-skating obsession, I heard a story on the radio about a skater I had watched in the past, Ekaterina Gordeeva. Her husband and figure-skating partner, Sergei Grinkov, died suddenly while they were practicing a routine. He was lifting Ekaterina high into the air when he dropped to the ice with a heart attack. I obsessed over the story for weeks. I waited expectantly during the six o'clock news for the sports update, hoping for new information on Ekaterina's loss. I filled pages and pages with my own retelling of the story, and wrote about how heartbroken I was for her. Janet found my writing one night and laughed at how ridiculous I was for being so invested in a story about two Russian skaters I had never met. I quickly grabbed my pages back, feigning an aloofness by crumpling them and casually tossing them aside, but I felt as though a deeply hidden part of me had been exposed.

When I was eleven, I became obsessed with a book called *Joni: An Unforgettable Story*, an autobiography by a young woman who became paralyzed after diving into a shallow lake and striking her head on the bottom. She writes about the weeks in the hospital that followed her accident, how frustrated she was by her inability to move, and how she finally came to accept her life that came after. I picked up the book daily, rereading the part about her accident, until I no longer needed the book in my hands to remember her words. Even today, as I recount the book that captivated me in my youth, I remember every part of Joni's story as if the accident had happened to me.

This trend, my fascination with the painful side of the human experience, continued throughout my life, acting as a counterweight to my own personal experiences, which remained sunny and bright until my late twenties. When Joey and I rented a small, ground-level apartment of our own in Edmonton, I became enthralled with a blog written by a woman named Tre, who had unexpectedly become a widow at thirty-three. Like Ekaterina, her husband had a heart attack, but Tre's husband had died in their bed and not on the ice.

One evening, I was reading Tre's most recent blog post, my left hand covering my mouth as I scrolled the screen of my laptop. It was in the middle of an intense Edmonton heat wave, and all of our patio doors and windows were open in an attempt to cool our loft-style flat, leaving me exposed to anyone walking by on the sidewalk. As my eyes wet with tears, I heard a voice yell, "Hey! You need to cheer up!" I looked up, startled, and I saw two men around my age standing on the sidewalk a few feet away. They were looking right at me. I wiped my face hurriedly, turning away from their intrusive gaze, and the laughter that followed while they walked away filled me with more shame than I'd have felt if I had been caught watching porn. Porn, at least, would have been understood. My longing to feel so close to the bereaved was much less explicable.

Perhaps my body, imprinted with an imperfect womb since birth, drove me to find fascination and beauty in loss, because without other people's stories to guide me through my many miscarriages, I would have been completely lost. Had my body been trying to tell me, all this time, that I would need to prepare for the ways it would bring pain into my life? Was it whispering to me all along, trying to tell me something was wrong?

Not long after the night in my apartment, I began a career that grants me entry to the most intimate lesson on grief. As a pediatric nurse, I am witness to some of the deepest moments of pain we can imagine as humans. After a child dies, grief fills a hospital room with its suffocating presence. It creeps up my neck as I listen to the sounds that follow. The wails of a devastated mother, the uttering of *No, no, no* by a father, and the silence of a chest. My tears fall readily, sobs escaping my throat, while I wash a small body with warm water, making sure the temperature is just right. I dress them, sliding lifeless limbs into pajamas and onesies, wrapping them in soft blankets before I gently lift the still-warm body of a child from their bed, and place them in the arms of their bereft mother. I put my hand tenderly on the child's forehead, caring for them as much in death as I did in life. It is a privilege to bear witness to these moments and to participate in such a sacred part of life: dying. As a nurse, I was dipping my toes into the cold waters of shock and despair and I had no idea that, all along, I was preparing for my own plunge into the frigidness of grief.

I now have a shelf in my library filled with books written by husbands who lost their wives, fathers who lost their small children, and an intense memoir written by a woman who lost her entire family in a tsunami. I have books about stillbirths and miscarriages, a book that even takes place within the four walls of the NICU where my son spent weeks of his early life. They are about loss and grief and the tenderest of hearts who have lost something big.

It's the place I retreat to when I am red-eyed and sleep-deprived. I am like Teddy, running my hands over the spines of books like his hands grazing the skin of my breasts. It's where you can find me on my darkest hours. Standing, or sitting cross-legged, on the hardwood floors of my small library, with books opened around me to pages that are underlined and dog-eared for this occasion. Their words are a release for the pain I am feeling. They are the place I go to find my reflection, and where I no longer feel alone. These words have gotten me out of bed on the toughest of days. They have carried me down the stairs to put on a pot of coffee and make breakfast for my son. They've given me a place to turn when I lacked the faith of a conventional religion. They became my religion. My source of hope amid despair. To give me the space to cry and laugh and to say to myself, *Yes, that's exactly what it's like.* They've allowed me to believe that perhaps what I have been given to bear is not as unbearable as I once thought. That I can still live with hope in my heart instead of anger, and how that is something I *can* control. The words that people have so generously given me have allowed me to believe that perhaps I, too, can be as resilient as they have been. I need to try.

21

▼

It is late March, and sunlight filters in through the blinds in Heather's office. I welcome the late-afternoon brightness, especially when compared to the dark winter day of our first appointment. The weather isn't the only thing in transition. I no longer feel a surge of adrenaline when I open the door to Heather's office. I am more relaxed in her presence, and I only shed a couple of tears during our previous session.

"Who are you most angry with?" Heather asks me after she sits in her chair. We often skip pleasantries and dive right in. It was jarring at first, but I am now used to the way she bluntly asks me questions I have never before considered.

"I'm not sure," I reply, thinking I am just angry. Isn't that the second phase of grief? Do I have to be angry *at* someone?

"Sometimes it can be hard to tell who we are angry with when we are grieving. Sometimes we are angry at nobody in particular, but sometimes we hold anger for people or things in our life. It can be an important step toward healing if you can determine where your anger is being directed."

Heather hands me a sheet of paper. It has a number of questions with lines underneath for my answers and a large empty circle in the centre. "I want you to fill this out before next week. This circle," she says, pointing, "represents all the anger you have. I want you to divide it into sections and give each one a title. It's a way for you to label your anger, to find its source, so you can move forward."

Heather always uses words like *healing* and *moving forward*, two things I never believed I could do.

I tuck the page into the black backpack I carry everywhere with me. It holds my notebook filled with all of Heather's assignments, the green leather journal I write in, and reminders of my son: toy cars, a spare diaper, wipes, and leftover Goldfish crackers crushed at the bottom. I leave with an eagerness to complete this task.

My next session is the following week, during my lunch break. I walk the few blocks to Heather's office, and I am caught in a downpour. The kind that leaves your hair soaked as if you've just stepped out of the shower. I go into the bathroom to dry off and notice all of the pages in my notebook have gotten wet. Turns out my backpack isn't waterproof. I pull them out, trying to dry them under the hand dryer to preserve what I had written. The ink has run slightly, giving the words a haziness around their edges, as though I have taken off my glasses.

I sit on Heather's couch and hand her my homework, expecting praise for having completed the assignment so diligently. The sheet is still damp, and the edges curl slightly in Heather's hands as she reads. After a painful minute, during which I study her face for any signs of approval, she says, "What you've written is quite interesting, Joanne."

Interesting isn't the word I am looking for; I wonder how I could have gotten the assignment wrong. She lays the sheet out on the distressed coffee table, smoothing the slightly crinkled edges to make them lay flat. I grab my cardboard coffee cup—I am always forgetting my reusable one—and peer over to see what she is talking about. I look at the pie chart I've filled in from the empty circle in the middle of the page. The chart that illustrates the anger I feel over my miscarriages. I look at Heather, still unsure what she finds so interesting.

"Look here," she says, pointing to the largest area I had drawn. It takes up seventy-five percent of the entire circle. She taps lightly with her neatly trimmed, oval fingernail, and continues. "You wrote here that you are most angry at your body. That's a lot of self-directed anger." I nod, finally seeing with clarity what she noticed. She sits back in her chair while I take a slow sip of my coffee.

When I set out to do the assignment days earlier, it made sense to feel angry at my body. It is my body that has failed me the most, so I blame it more than anyone or anything. I didn't realize I cannot separate myself from my body. We are the same. My body that has failed me, and my mind that is hurting. I didn't realize, until that moment, that when I am screaming in my car with anger, I am screaming at myself.

"You have incredibly high expectations for yourself," Heather continues; I notice she does not phrase it as a question as she normally does. We've now spent a number of weeks together and she seems confident in her assessment of who I am.

I tell her how earlier in the week my son threw a temper tantrum. The kind two-year-olds are notorious for. Something innocuous set him off. Perhaps he was hungry or tired, or simply felt frustrated that I wouldn't let him play dangerously on the stairs in our home. He erupted with anger. His face turned red and he screamed and thrashed and threw himself on the ground. I snapped. I sat him back up and yelled at him to stop it. His eyes grew wide, as I don't typically yell. I instantly felt terrible. I embraced him tightly, whispering "I'm so sorry" into his ear.

After he went to bed, I wrote in my journal through tears. *I am a horrible mother*, I wrote. *I've for sure messed him up for life.* I feel guilty even days later. I'm not sure I know of any parents who haven't snapped at their children at least once, and I would never think twice to see a friend react the same way with her child. *Motherhood is hard*, I would think, smiling in her direction while she tried to calm a raging child. I am unable to speak to myself in the same way. I can forgive everyone else for their imperfections, but I am unable to let myself be anything other than perfect. The perfect mom, the perfect wife, the perfect woman.

The same goes for my miscarriages. I am unable to look past any tiny misstep I took during my pregnancies, and along with blaming myself, I feel angry that I am never able to meet my own impossible expectations. I turn on myself, quickly and easily, something I have done my entire life.

"Why do you expect yourself to be perfect?" Heather asks me.

I shrug. "I've always been this way." I wonder when Freud is going to come into the conversation.

When I was younger, I berated myself for seemingly innocent things. I was a Highland dancer for many years as a girl, wearing a kilt and performing on stage to bagpipe music. When I was fourteen, our dance group was hired for a wedding reception being held in an old barn converted into a dining hall. The bride used to be a dancer and wanted to incorporate her love of the Scottish tradition. It was August and we arrived at the outdoor ceremony early in the evening. We hadn't been invited to the actual wedding—we were the entertainment and not guests, after all—so we all convened behind the barn where we heard clinking glasses, loud voices, and music coming from inside.

The mosquitoes were gnawing at my exposed skin. I kept swatting them away, but I ended up with large red welts on my knees and elbows anyway. They must have been attracted to the sweet-smelling hairspray that was holding my hair tight in its French braid. Our bagpiper hadn't shown up yet, but once he did, our show would begin. We stood in small circles, twelve girls, giggling and laughing together. Our moms stood back, chatting amongst themselves, one of them occasionally reaching over to push in a bobby pin or tuck a stray piece of hair behind an ear.

Soon, a car pulled up and parked in the driveway a few metres from where we stood. We all looked to see a man step out from the passenger side. He was wearing a green kilt, with a furry sporran hanging loose around his hips, looking like an old-timey fanny pack. He put his hat on as soon as he stood. His movements looked odd, unnatural even. He felt the edge of the open door, patting its side like a police officer searching for weapons, stopping when his fingers touched the handle. He gently pushed the door closed with a quiet click. I was so accustomed to the way my friends and siblings slammed car doors shut it felt disconcerting to see someone treat one with such tenderness. When he turned around, I looked at the man's face and I saw a cloudy dullness in his eyes.

The driver, a man who appeared to be the same age as the bagpiper, stepped around from the driver's side of the car. He took the man's elbow, guiding him toward our group. The bagpiper was blind.

He introduced himself as Andrew. We all mumbled hello and I could barely look away from those milky eyes that never looked in our direction. I was curious, since I had never before spent time with anyone who had a visual impairment, and his ability to move about was fascinating. His friend handed him his bagpipes. Andrew gave the belly a few pumps, blowing into the mouthpiece, creating a low hum that indicated the instrument was ready. He placed the instrument confidently under his left arm. He appeared nervous—or was I just nervous around him?—and I felt my heart warm toward him. I was filled with a strong desire to put him at ease. I wanted him to know I saw him, that I could see him for more than his impairment. I wanted to say something, but I felt awkward and self-conscious. I didn't want to come across as condescending toward the man. I was afraid I might say the wrong thing.

We heard the MC in the barn announce it was time for the show to start, and our moms shushed us, telling us it was time to go on. We assumed a straight line like young soldiers, pasting smiles on our faces, and we skipped into the middle of the barn. The bagpiper was led to the edge of the stage by his friend. We danced for half an hour and after we raced off the stage, we all stood chatting, laughing about our missteps and zippers that had come undone, before it was time to go home. The bagpiper stood quietly on the outer edge of our group, not saying anything, while his friend packed up their car. I occasionally looked over at him, wanting to say something, but never did.

When I got home that night, I turned to my diary to sort out my feelings. *Why didn't I speak to him?* I wrote. *He would have been so much more comfortable if only I had said something to him. I am a rotten person.* I wrote three pages worth of self-abuse, my anger toward myself steaming off the page. I dwelled on my missed opportunity to have a human connection with the bagpiper, assuming so many things were wrong with me that had stopped me from doing so.

I belittle myself for doing things that make me human. I demand perfection and I always let myself down because it is an unattainable goal. With my miscarriages, it feels as though I have the biggest reason of all to hate myself.

"We're going to work on this," Heather says gently. "The first step is recognizing our faults. We can't change anything we don't acknowledge."

I look at my hands, uncertain. I don't know if I can let go of my deep-seeded belief that I can somehow change who I am if I try hard enough. That I am capable of the one thing humans are incapable of: perfection. I don't know how to let go of who I've always wanted to be and allow myself the freedom of being.

22

▼

"I WANT TO HAVE A SECOND CHILD BEFORE MY SON GETS TOO comfortable being an only child," a friend tells me. We are having coffee together, our sons playing beside each other, still too young to play with one another.

"I get what you mean," I say, looking away briefly. I don't tell her I am still going through my fourth miscarriage and that my dream of having children close in age is being flushed down the toilet daily. I can't blame her for a seemingly harmless comment. Had she been sitting with most of her other mom friends, they would have likely all agreed and discussed the merits of siblings who are close in age. Had my life gone differently, I would have said the exact same thing, thought nothing of it.

I, too, used to think all of this was in my control. I used to think that positive pregnancy tests meant a beautiful baby. My friend lives in a world where she can control how, and when, she has children. I live in a world where there are a dozen possible outcomes to a single event. On the outside I look exactly like her, but she is the before version, who I could have been.

I don't see her again for many months, not because what she said had hurt me so much but because I struggle to fit in with a lot of my mom friends in the months after my fourth miscarriage. Almost every time I hang out with other moms, I excuse myself for a few moments alone because I feel like I can't quite relate.

The women who ask me how I am doing are my saviours. I need them intensely, acting like an uninvited houseguest, outstaying my welcome. I give details when none are asked for and I speak at length, even as these friends grow uncomfortable. Some are gracious and let me talk as much as I need to, and others get bored and the conversation fizzles. The people who know what I am going through and don't say anything to me about it are harder on my heart. To have my loss unacknowledged by them is deeply painful. I forgive them, and I understand their ignorance, because before I experienced anything like this, I would have likely done the same.

It feels like each loss is a secret meant to be kept, something shameful to be hidden from view. I perpetuate the silence by pretending to be okay, and I sometimes shut down when people try talking to me about it. I open up to strangers sitting in a waiting room, but not to my mom. My boss at work, but not my sister. Perhaps I feel less vulnerable opening up to people who are more acquaintances than friends. I am embarrassed by my pain and I don't want to appear ungrateful for what I have, even though I am so sad about what I have lost.

Very few people have seen my naked grief, the unmasked version of myself. I keep it tucked away, protected from platitudes or judgment from others. I hold it closely, building a wall around it, letting few see what I carry. I am told that I am strong, that I am resilient, that they can't imagine what I have endured. But I am simply trying to hide my weakest part from view, hoping it won't break me irreparably. I am trying to fit a wooden ship into a glass bottle, a task that feels impossible.

I DECIDE TO TAKE SOME TIME AWAY TO HEAL BEFORE JOEY AND I plan for the future. I book another miscarriage trip to England to visit a dear friend, Jenny, whom I've known for fourteen years. This time, I know my grief will be coming along for the ride. It is my first big trip away from my son, and I cry when I walk into the security line and can no longer see his arms waving at me. I feel his absence when I sit, undisturbed, at the gate, reading a book and drinking a hot coffee. It feels luxurious to have so much uninterrupted time to myself, and yet when I look at the families with small children nearby, I want to reach out and say, *I'm like you, too.*

I spend a long weekend in London. Jenny and I eat delicious food, speak about our lives, and share her bed in her beautiful London flat like we are teenagers again, sharing secrets late into the night. We spend time together with an ease that comes with having someone in your life for so long. I admit to Jenny that I feel lost and don't know what will happen next as we stroll the beautiful streets of London. It is uplifting and sad and wonderful all at the same time.

When I return home, Joey and I decide we want to try and get pregnant again. My trip, which Joey encouraged me to take, gave me some time to grieve, and when I return, we are both still hopeful for another child. We have not yet spoken aloud what we are both fearing most of all: that another child may never be born. In the evenings, once more, after Teddy is in bed, we speak with certainty of the family we will have, not letting any doubts of a second child pass between our lips. We calculate the months it may take us to get pregnant, discussing when we will likely have our second baby, the sibling for our son. My ovulation tests tell me I am ovulating, and we make love, neither of us admitting how terrified we are.

Two weeks later, on the day my period is set to arrive, I wake with an almost imperceptible tenderness in my breasts. I pace around my house, unsettled that the telltale symptoms of my period have not yet arrived. By the afternoon, I can't wait any longer. My sister is visiting, so I tell her I need to buy limes for supper, and I drive to the nearest store, leaving Teddy to play with his beloved aunt.

I lock myself in the grimy bathroom of the grocery store.
Pregnant.

I take five deep breaths before I shakily walk back to my car, forgetting the limes on the edge of the stained porcelain sink. I sit for a few minutes in the car, the pregnancy test perched on my lap, and I wonder what we are going to do. It doesn't feel like the right time to have another miscarriage. It never will. I do some quick math in my head and realize this child would arrive in March. Our children would be three years apart. A number that feels perfect.

Back at home, I admit to my sister where I went. I've never been good at lying, especially about important things. While running my hands through my hair, mirroring Joey's mannerisms, I tell her I'm pregnant.

Instead of a well-planned announcement to Joey, I go outside to sit on the front step, knowing he will be home soon. I feel like I'm twelve again, waiting with my younger brother after we broke my parents' bed after playing on it. We decided to face my mom when she got home from work, knowing it was better to get our punishment over with than to wait. When she pulled up, she saw both of us sitting on the front stoop, our heads bowed, knowing we were about to get grounded.

When Joey pulls up, he steps out of the car and I give him a little wave from where I sit.

"What's going on?" he asks.

"Sit."

He sits beside me, and I hand him the positive test. He puts his arm around me and squeezes. I put my head on his shoulder. We don't say anything in those few minutes, just sit looking at the flowers in our front yard, listening to my sister playing with our son inside. His laughter engulfs us, while we dare to hope for more.

I HAVE A NEW DOCTOR, A SPECIALIST WHO DEALS WITH problematic women like myself, and when first meeting him, several weeks before Joey and I sat on our front porch, I tell him how I am willing to subject myself to anything he can offer to have another child. I am looking for him to give me a magic cure, an answer as to why this has been so hard. He gives me neither.

He says how it's unusual for a woman like me to have so much trouble. Women with heart-shaped uteruses conceive and give birth all the time. I am the worst case he's ever seen. I am, apparently, unlucky.

"I think I have less than a ten percent chance of helping you, Joanne. We could do one small exploratory surgery, but it's unlikely to help."

I nod my head, having heard this before, and smile in response to such poor odds, but my arms wrap themselves tightly around my stomach, and my legs cross in an attempt to protect myself from the shrapnel of his words.

"What do you want?" he asks, interrupting my anxious silence.

"I want another child," I reply, laughing nervously, trying to keep the desperation from my voice.

"I can't guarantee you anything. Nobody can." It's clear he isn't in the business of handing out false hope.

"I'm willing to do anything, even if the chances of success are small." I pause a moment, considering if it is safe to say what comes next. "These four miscarriages haven't been easy." My voice breaks and I swallow. "I would like to know there is a chance, even if it's small."

He scribbles some notes in my chart and I fill the silence like I do with Heather.

"Have you ever seen anyone like me before? What happened to them?"

"Well, you haven't even seen how bad it can be. I had a patient, similar to you, who lost one baby at twenty weeks and her second at twenty-two weeks. She decided it was too painful to try again after that."

I inhale sharply and my lungs fill with the pain that woman must have felt. I allow myself to imagine if that were me. *How brave*, I think. *How brave to have tried, to have tried again, and how brave of her to stop.*

"I'm here because I'm not done trying yet. If you think there is a small chance that another surgery might help, I am all in."

"Okay. I can't make any promises that this operation will be of any use to you, but let's see what we can see." He says a date out loud, and I pull out the calendar on my phone, making a quick note that reads *Surgery Day* for the middle of July.

He asks if I plan to keep trying to conceive while I wait for the surgery, which is three months away. I nod my head, unable to consider a time when I wouldn't be trying to have a baby. He scribbles on a pink pad of paper. If I am to get pregnant, I will take three different prescriptions: a daily injection filled with a blood thinner, a blood thinner to take orally, and the same hormones Dr. Comeau prescribed years earlier to try and prevent another miscarriage. After ripping off the prescriptions from his pad, he reminds me that none of these have shown any evidence of working for anyone like me. I take them anyway, hoping they hold the magic cure I came here for.

"Good luck," he says, pushing the stool back under the desk. "I'll see you in a couple of months." He leaves the room to tend to another patient. I leave the office with my prescriptions in hand and the dismal odds of having another baby.

The week of my scheduled surgery, I discover I am pregnant.

I frantically call my doctor's office, asking to be seen immediately. With my surgery cancelled, I crane my neck during an early ultrasound to see my five-week-old baby on a black-and-white screen.

"Everything looks good," my doctor says, covering me with a sheet. "Let's hope things continue to go well."

23

▼

I TAKE MY PREGNANCY COCKTAIL LIKE CLOCKWORK EVERY DAY and I feel like a pregnancy junkie. A woman addicted to the idea of babies, willing to roll up my sleeves and tap my veins with a persistent *thwap* to make it happen. I lift my shirt, holding the fabric beneath my chin, and expose my bruised and bloated belly. I look for an area that is not as tender as others, and I breathe in the sterile scent of the alcohol swab, wiping in circular motions on the skin I intend to jab. I remove the rubber top covering the needle with my teeth and, while pinching a flab of skin and tissue, I plunge the needle into the delicate spot on my stomach. Without taking a breath, I inject the burning liquid into my body, pushing down on the plunger until the syringe is empty. I exhale as the needle recoils on its own, and I apply pressure with a cotton swab to dull the burning that continues for over a minute. I ritualistically clean the area and place the needle among its peers in a locked storage box tucked away in the bowels of my bathroom closet. I appreciate the routine of it all. The injection generates a pain filled with relief. Perhaps it's akin to running a razor blade down the length of your arm, releasing yourself from demons much worse than any physical pain.

The summer of my sixth pregnancy passes in a blur of injections, doctor's appointments, and fear so intense I wake gasping for air in the middle of the night. I fight against my instinct to attach to this new life growing inside me because it is too painful to consider it might not survive. Joey and I barely speak about the baby in those early weeks. We don't even allow ourselves to use our *ifs* and *mights*. We try to survive by pretending I am not pregnant.

There are shadowy thoughts of a big pregnant belly or a sibling who looks like Teddy, but I allow them to pass like a leaf floating on a river. I don't let myself think about being pregnant as soon as I wake. Instead, I push the thoughts aside, filling my head with to-do lists and meal-planning, anything to silence their persistence. I stop looking at calendars and refuse to estimate how pregnant I will be when I attend our friend's wedding in September. I don't want to have a date on the calendar circled, even if only in my mind. I think that by eliminating the joy I can avoid its dark counterpart.

I begin to bleed at seven weeks.

I am alone in an ultrasound room, waiting to see if my baby is alive. I can picture it all. The first separation of the embryo that has attached itself to my womb. The small specks of blood forming at the corner that lift off, like a scab being picked by a fingernail. The small gummy bear–shaped baby folding in on itself. Perhaps it will have already been dead before it began. My uterus will tense and pulse and more and more of it will get ripped away. Blood will pour out. From the placenta, from the space behind it, from the baby itself. It will come out in a gush. And another. And then another. It will shudder and rip apart anything inside. It will come out in clumps and bits of tissue. The entire wall of my uterus will separate, resulting in an eruption that cannot be abated. I imagine all of this happening while I am waiting for the confirmation that this baby has also died.

"I've lost four," I say to the ultrasound tech, trying to explain why I am shaking so badly on the bed. She asks if I am cold, but I shake my head. "These ultrasounds are pretty traumatic for me." I explain.

"I understand," she says softly, zooming in on the baby we both know is in grave danger. After only a couple of seconds passes, she announces, "There's the heartbeat." I see the flicker that I have been straining my eyes to see. I erupt in sobs, making the rest of the scan impossible to complete, the type of crying that comes from the bottom of your feet and leaves you breathless as you try to stop it. The tech puts her hand on my arm, trying to reassure me this was not another miscarriage and that there is nothing that can explain my bleeding, but I cannot stop crying. She gives me a few minutes in the room alone to collect myself as much as possible before I make my way past a waiting room filled with women who are likely wondering why such sadness could be heard coming from room four.

After the scan, I go home and cry in Joey's arms. Tears of relief that our baby is still alive, but of terror for this child who now has a heartbeat. Although I have tried to remain unattached to this baby, the ultrasound stripped away any ability to appear aloof. I can no longer deny myself the truth that has always been there. I will do anything to keep this baby.

My doctor phones me that afternoon, and he gives me no suggestions on what I can do differently. I suggest bedrest, more hormones, and I quote a study I found on the internet. He tells me there is nothing that can be done. I am certain a light breeze could cause me to miscarry and I wonder how I will sustain this level of stress for another seven months.

The weeks pass and my pants grow tight; somehow, I am still pregnant. I keep up my daily injections and my stomach is spotted with dark bruises as a result. The self-abuse is therapeutic, as it allows me to believe I am doing something. I pretend like I have control and I forget every lesson I have learned with Heather. I have avoided seeing her ever since I got pregnant, cancelling each appointment because I am too afraid of being forced to see the truth. I do not want to relinquish my perceived sense of control because it feels like the only thing keeping me steady. This magical belief that I am in control is a touchstone, my lucky rabbit's foot, a way for me to cope with the anxiety of it all. I do none of the homework she's given me to focus on in times of stress. I stop writing, reading, or trying to think too deeply. Instead, I fill my evenings with mindless television, allowing myself to consider that perhaps this baby will make it if only I can move slowly, unassumingly, and tiptoe gently through the world.

It is the end of August and I am approaching the twelfth week of pregnancy, the golden week, the week that allows most women to relax into their current state, assured by their ability to make it through the high-risk first trimester. It is the week of carefully planned pregnancy announcements and congratulatory messages being shared by all

Just before the golden week arrives, I start bleeding again.

After waiting nervously in the emergency department for another ultrasound, Joey and I look with wonder at the screen when the doctor walks us through what she is seeing: a baby the size of a lime, its arms and legs waving to us from the blackened screen of the monitor. A darkened area is also on the screen, tucked in the corner opposite our baby. It is described to us as a blood clot of unknown origin, and it is producing symptoms that are a red herring for another miscarriage.

Joey snaps a photo of the baby on his phone. And when I look at it, I feel as though I am staring directly into the sun. Months later, I pull the photo out to look at its profile, its button nose, and the lips that remind me of my son's. I have memorized its every detail, and I can sometimes imagine their scent when I look at their picture. The sickly-sweet smell of newborns, a mixture of earth and milk and something you can't quite place, like the secret ingredient in your grandmother's cookie recipe.

When I am twelve weeks pregnant, less than a week after that photo is taken, I wake early after having an unsettling dream. I dreamed the baby had died. I put my hands on my stomach and feel cramps that are different than before. I lie as still as I can, trying to decipher if I am imagining them because of the dream. I roll over to reach for the bottle of hormones I take twice daily, and I feel a slight gush of fluid I instinctively know is my water breaking.

I lie on my back quietly, trying not to move. I tell myself this can't happen this early, there's no way, water doesn't break at twelve weeks. I must be imagining it. Minutes later I stand, and another gush. Even in my state of denial, I know what is happening. My heart is pounding. I had experienced this with my son, the inexplicable, innate understanding that I am in labour. I walk to the bathroom and inspect the carnage of my now soaked-through underwear and pajama bottoms. I feel panic creep up my neck. I can't breathe. I am suffocating with grief already. My unborn child is dying.

I sob when I sit in the chair at triage. I tell the nurse it sounds unbelievable, but my water has broken at three months.

"Is this your first pregnancy?" she asks, typing on her computer.

"Sixth," I reply shakily. "I've had four miscarriages in the past."

"Oh my," she says, looking at me with concern. She silently hands me some tissues and tells me it won't be long.

I ask to see the ultrasound. The tech looks at me; she is young, and I remember being that young and green in a profession that deals with life and death. Your life experience is limited, and you are often unsure what to do when faced with a question like that. She is not allowed to tell me the results, even though her silence and persistence over my abdomen have been telling, and she waffles over whether or not I should see what she has seen. I gently push. "I know you can't tell me anything, but please, show me the screen."

She reluctantly flips the monitor to a still image of my baby and my stomach lurches. I feel sick. It has lost its protective sac of water, the one thing allowing it to grow unencumbered in my uterus, and the fluid with which it needs to develop its lungs and other major organs. The baby is no longer floating in a sea of black. You can barely discern the baby from my uterus, the technology unable to distinguish my flesh from theirs. I see a red number above the baby indicating their heartbeat, and I know they are still alive. But I also know they will not survive.

"Thank you," I reply meekly, not looking her in the eye, wishing I hadn't looked.

A doctor quietly tells me the baby will likely die soon. "Is there anyone I can call?" he asks, sitting on the edge of my bed. I shake my head, unable to speak. I need to get home to Joey. To the safety of his arms. I pick up my bag and leave.

At home, Joey and I curl up together, crying, unable to say any words that might bring comfort to each other. My uterus feels like a morgue. I have so much to apologize for. My body is crushing our baby, and it is unbearable to know this.

In the hours after my water breaks, I place my hands on my stomach, trying to pass something that might resemble comfort to the fetus who is dying inside. They are struggling to move; their cord will eventually suffocate them before they ever take a breath. I don't want them to be afraid. I don't know how to comfort my child, though, when it is me who is hurting them.

I'm sorry.

I'm sorry.

I'm sorry.

That night I feel the cramps I intuitively know are the last signs of life from my dying baby. I cling to the edge of my sink in my bathroom while the contractions squeeze my abdomen like a boa constrictor trying to kill its prey. I try to send the last messages of love and kindness to the child I will never meet. I walk around the hallways of my house, trying not to picture their decomposing body because I know what decomposing bodies look like. I know how pink flesh turns to dark purple and then to black after a heartbeat stops.

THE NEXT DAY, I AM IN MY DOCTOR'S OFFICE, WAITING TO SEE if my baby has given up its fight or if I have to make the unbearable decision to undergo an abortion to end their suffering. My kind, lovely doctor places a probe over the side of my body where the baby had landed. He spends a few seconds looking around and he pauses where we should be able to see a beating heart. He stops and we wait. There are no playful limbs like before. There is no red number indicating they are still alive. The monitor is silent. The image is still.

"I don't think there is a heartbeat," he says gently. "It should be right here."

My eyes well with tears. They are not only tears of sadness, but also tears of relief. Relief that my baby's suffering is over. Relief that I won't have to kill them in a more brutal way than my body had already chosen to. Relief that I no longer have to fear the baby's death, because they have already died.

I sob for a minute while my doctor sits beside my bed, and I explain how even though I am sad, I am relieved it is over. I tell him how I have been hoping there wouldn't be a heartbeat, as hard as that is to admit.

"That's what I had been thinking too," he replies, and he wipes the jelly off my stomach, the monitor turning black.

I sit, wiping the tears that have pooled around my neck and ears, and I pause for a moment, trying to gather the strength to discuss what is to come next.

"So," I start, "do you think there is anything you can do for someone like me? It seems like all of these are my fault. You need three things to have a pregnancy go well: a uterus capable of providing space for a fetus to grow, an umbilical cord that can deliver it nutrients, and a baby who is healthy. If it weren't for my uterus, this baby would have been fine. I'm the missing one-third of the equation."

My doctor looks at me kindly and says, "That's not fair to put this on yourself. You have had an incredibly hard time. Even when a pregnancy goes well for you, it doesn't exactly go well. Maybe it's time we discuss using a gestational carrier." He glances at my chart, looking to confirm my age. I am thirty-three. That looming fertile window is closing. "If it's something you want to do, we need to look at doing this before you are thirty-five. Your chances decrease dramatically after that."

As I mourn the loss of my sixth baby, I calculate in my head that I have about a year and a half to decide whether or not to freeze a bundle of eggs, should I ever wish to have another baby.

24

▼

I TEXT MY FRIEND JENNY TO TELL HER I LOST THE BABY. She phones me right away even though the time distance means it is late in the UK. I feel guilty, knowing she has to work early the next day. After picking up, I tell her my well-rehearsed speech about how it isn't entirely unexpected considering my past and how lucky I feel to have Teddy. When I am done, the phone goes silent for a moment.

"You're not a failure, Joanne," Jenny says softly. Even though an ocean separates us physically, the distance shrinks with her words. It feels as though she is sitting in the room beside me.

I stifle a sob.

"I know," I reply, my voice raising as I trail off, as though I am asking a question.

"No, really," she continues. "You are not a failure."

I let her hear me cry. My shoulders relax since I no longer have to pretend to be anything other than sad.

I sit on the edge of my bed. "But I am." I look out my bedroom window at the trees and the ocean that line my backyard.

"I know you think that," she says. "I just had to say it anyway."

I AM WAITING FOR MY SURGEON TO ARRIVE. MY VIEW OF THE OR ceiling is hauntingly familiar. A nurse connects me to a cardiac monitor, and I don't respond to her small talk about the hurricane on its way. I am tucked inside my head, trying to remember who I am, but I keep coming up short. I don't know who I am if I am not trying to make a baby, keep a baby, have a baby. Has my desire to procreate become a chronic disease I need to treat? While lying on the stretcher, I can smell the sour milk of a newborn's neck, the scent of diaper balm, pink baby lotion. There is no baby here; my mind is creating things I want to be true.

I feel like I am on fire. A rush of heat travels up my arm, dissipating in my chest as a doctor pushes the milky white anesthetic into my IV. A mask is placed over my mouth and nose. The oxygen smells strangely chemical, like plastic, and nothing like air. I blink and it's dark.

Joey is holding my clammy hand, and I feel worse than I remember feeling after any of my past surgeries. Perhaps because this baby had made it further along, it will take me longer to recover physically. Or perhaps losing so many is taking an even more devastating toll. My nurse gives me an extra dose of analgesic, noticing my rapid breaths, and I try to go back to sleep. The dark nothing of surgery was a relief but I am unable to slip back into its comforting void.

"How old is your son?" my nurse asks.

"He's two," I say, opening my eyes, and I smile. Joey squeezes my hand and gives a tiny smile too. "All of this," I wave my arms around the recovery room to indicate my current situation, "is showing me just how lucky we are to have him." It is a knee-jerk response to use my son as a splint against my pain. My attempt to put others at ease by hiding behind the armour of his existence.

My nurse looks up seriously from her page and says, "You don't have to say that. It's good to be grateful, but you don't have to say that right now."

I put down my armour, allowing myself to be unprotected, vulnerable. I am sad. I am the saddest I have ever been. Most people want to hear how grateful and appreciative I am to be a mother because it makes them more comfortable in my presence. I've learned to sandwich any discussion about my miscarriages with *but I have a son*, to put others at ease. My recovery room nurse has read my encyclopedia-sized chart riddled with complications, diagnoses, tests, and the outline of my dead babies in sequential order. She is accepting my sadness in its uninhibited form, not demanding a more palatable version.

She cares for me without making small talk. She helps me into my mesh underwear and pad, gives me pills that I take with sips of cold water from a thimble-sized cup. My throat feels like sandpaper. When I'm allowed to leave, she hugs me tightly and when we pull away, she puts her hands on my shoulders.

"I'll be thinking of you, Joanne," she says, and I see a wetness in her eyes as she squeezes my shoulders. I believe her.

HURRICANE DORIAN HITS THE NEXT DAY. I WAKE TO A MENACING grey sky and the rain arrives by mid-morning. Our lights flicker twice, and we lose power. Branches fall with a sickening crack near our living room windows and Teddy runs around the house with a headlamp on, enjoying the excitement of the storm. I sit stoically on the couch for much of the day, far away in my mind.

Joey and I didn't prepare for the storm, since I only got home from recovery hours before it hit. We listened to the radio on the way back from the hospital with announcers reminding us what to do, but we didn't bother to check our flashlights for batteries and our pantry is nearly bare by the time the power goes out. Joey and I eat crackers and cheese for lunch. We let Teddy eat cereal by the handful. I barely register the intensity of the storm, my inner turmoil stronger than a category 2 hurricane.

Late afternoon falls and our home is in the eye of the storm. The rain and wind stop. The air is full of energy, the kind where you can sense the storm will return in a matter of minutes. It is a tired metaphor for how I feel. We put on our raincoats and boots and the three of us go outside. Teddy is taken by all the fallen trees in our yard, and we marvel at how many leaves are stuck to the side of our wooden house. It reminds us of the puzzle pieces we lay out on the floor earlier to pass the time. How when we first tipped the box upside down, the pieces landed in disarray. We see shingles in our front yard that have blown off the roof, and we look to where a split tree branch dangles precariously above our deck. Soon the rain picks up again and we retreat back inside.

The next morning is sunny and bright, and I find myself missing the storm. We wander outside to clean our yard, talking to our neighbours who had a tree fall on their house. It is angled awkwardly over their porch, the trim of their house dented by its heavy trunk. Everyone is safe, all family members accounted for. I place my hand over my bloated abdomen, wishing I could say the same. Joey and Teddy clean the yard while I go back to bed. I lie as still as I can, wishing for sleep.

Joey leaves for a business trip the following day. Though it has been planned for weeks, he debated cancelling after we lost the baby, but I insisted he go. "It's already gone, love," I told him. "There's nothing you can do." He leaves with a worried look on his face as I feign confidence in my ability to hold everything together until his return.

At suppertime, I take Teddy out to eat. Our power has not yet returned and the little amount of food we had in our pantry is mostly gone, except for a few tins of tuna and a package of noodles we can't cook. I don't dare open the fridge, which has long lost its ability to preserve anything inside. When we return home, I crawl into bed as soon as Teddy is asleep, exhausted from doing the bare necessities for us both.

The next day comes and our house remains dark. We make use of friends and family for showers, and all anyone talks about is the hurricane. I have nothing to contribute; I'm unable to think of anything except the baby. Everyone has a harrowing tale about fallen trees or cranes tumbling to the ground. I am left feeling like my baby hadn't mattered, as though its recognition is also a casualty of the storm.

I go back to work and my co-workers gasp that I am still without power, saying how terrible that must be. I shrug in response. I simply don't care. Losing power feels so inconsequential compared to everything else I am experiencing.

Damage to the power lines in our neighbourhood is extensive, and five days have now passed without electricity. Teddy never tires of our forced camping excursion; he is always up for an adventure, and he loves wearing his headlamp. Joey returns home that evening, and he hugs me tightly in our darkened foyer. I tell him I need to go for a walk and leave Joey to put Teddy to bed, feeling incapable of managing another bedtime. I click Maddy's leash onto her collar and walk outside.

Our neighbourhood is dark, the hum of generators filling the air with an unfamiliar buzz. I can see where trees have fallen and the docks that usually stand on the water have been forced ashore by the powerful surf. I pause at an inlet, watching the calm of the water that was so destructive days before. I listen to a foghorn while tears roll down my face.

When I return home, I can hear the sounds of Teddy's feet running around inside the house and his laughter wafts out of an open window. I can picture Joey chasing him around the house, trying to wrangle him into pajamas. I sit on our front stoop, petting Maddy who has crawled into my lap. I look at the trees that are now bare in our front yard. The naked branches look out of place for late summer, their green leaves usually still lush this time of year.

Maddy starts to bark. I try soothing her, but she is straining on the leash. A car has pulled off the road right in front of our house. I can't see it since our own vehicles are blocking my view. I hear a car door open and close. I look expectantly, wondering who could be visiting this time of night, and I see my friend Phil walking toward me.

"Hi buddy," he says, giving me a tiny wave.

Phil and his wife, Lisa, are two of our greatest friends. We met five years earlier, belonging to a group of four couples. Before we all had children, we held fancy three-course dinner parties, drank bottles of wine, and played games late into the night. Now, we order pizzas, drink cheap beers from the bottle, and let our kids chase each other from room to room while we try to squeeze in a conversation.

Phil and Lisa lost a baby, too.

"How are you doing?" he asks, reaching out his arms to give me a hug.

"Not great," I reply honestly, speaking into his chest. He nods and doesn't say anything for a moment.

"We brought you guys a little something. We know how awful this is." He hands me an envelope and I thank him through tear-filled eyes. We speak for a few minutes before he gets back into his car and drives away.

I sit on my stoop and open the envelope. There is a card with words of sympathy and kindness in Lisa's familiar handwriting and a gift certificate tucked inside for a local spa. I hold the card tightly against my chest and then walk back inside the house to show Joey what our dear friends have given us. I am so grateful for Lisa and Phil's kind gesture, for Phil showing up at the exact moment when I needed someone to recognize my pain. And he hadn't once asked me about the hurricane.

DAYS AFTER OUR POWER RETURNS, I STEP OUT OF THE SHOWER, looking at my leaking breasts and my swollen abdomen. I wonder what the current state of my body would be called. I put on a pair of hospital-issued mesh underwear that have become, to me, a symbol of motherhood. I tuck a pad inside that is more diaper than not. I'm not postpartum, I have no baby to hold, and yet I am not entirely unlike a woman who has just given birth. Our swollen bellies, the milk staining our shirts, the blurry-eyed discovery of ourselves in a territory unfamiliar. I am not them, but who am I? What am I? My arms are empty, but my abdomen juts out far enough to make people wonder, sometimes aloud, if I am pregnant. I wrap my towel tightly around my body again, trying to suppress the milk that wants to come. Even my body is confused by what it is.

I get dressed, wearing a loose-fitting shirt that covers any remaining signs of pregnancy, and I meet Joey and Teddy down-stairs. The three of us get in the car and Joey drives us to a suburb ten minutes away. I carefully get out of the car and walk up to a front door with balloons tied outside, the telltale sign that a child's birthday party is underway. I ring the doorbell, clutch-ing my son's hand for my own protection. The door opens and everything feels too bright and too quiet. My ears are ringing. I see people smiling and silent words forming on their lips. I hear somebody laugh. It sounds too high and too cartoonish to be real, and I discover it is my own. I walk through rooms filled with balloons and small children running around. Someone hands me a drink and I let the cold alcohol wake me from my stupor.

We gather in circles and talk about the banalities of life. I am asked the usual question in these social events—"So, what's new with you guys?"—and I can feel my fake smile fading. My hands shake slightly while I wrack my brain for something, anything, appropriate to say in this scenario. Anything that doesn't have to do with dying fetuses and premature water-breaking and surgeries and grief.

Joey sees me struggling to form words and he steps in to speak for the both of us, putting his hand on my back. "Oh, you know," he starts, "summer was busy, the usual." He is always more adept at managing his emotions over a miscarriage than I will ever be. His body is not consumed by the physical act of miscarrying. He is able to go about his day as normal without pausing during a painful contraction or needing to change pads hourly. He doesn't need to roll up his sleeves to give blood or take medication that gives him stomach ulcers. His grief is also different, less visceral, and more abstract than mine. He feels the pain deeply but compartmentalizes and moves forward in a way that's impossible for me to do.

The conversation shifts to recent sporting events and beach vacations past. I sit in the corner, relieved I don't have to speak.

I look around the room at the happy families surrounding me. Mothers breastfeeding infants, children asking for more cake, toddlers stumbling around aimlessly. Teddy, left to his own devices, is licking the icing off a cupcake like a Popsicle. I feel like a predator. I look at each woman wondering if she is done having children. *Has she had any complications?* I wonder. *Is her womb a safe place for babies to grow?* I am window-shopping for a uterus. A place I could put our tiny embryo and have it turn into a baby, because my body is no place to grow a child.

A MONTH AFTER THE HURRICANE I TAKE A QUIET WALK TO GET
the mail. It is after supper and before bedtime, an hour that
can sometimes feel like ten with a toddler. I want a bit of fresh
air and a few minutes alone. I step outside onto our wooden
porch, feeling the crisp evening air, and I pull my cardigan like a
blanket around me. I walk quietly to where the mailboxes stand
like guards along the side of the road. It's dark, and the gravel
crunches beneath my feet as I approach. I turn the key in the
lock, feeling the resistance of the cold metal. I open the door, its
hinges creaking as it swings open, and I see a small parcel tucked
inside. I haven't ordered anything, so I wonder who could have
sent me a package.

Smiling, I pull out the box, anticipating a gift from a friend. I
look at the label and a lump forms in my throat. It is from a baby
formula company. I stand in the cold, the door of my mailbox
flung wide open, and open a box decorated with a pattern of baby
bottles and rattles. I lift the cover and a small letter with a stock
photo of a baby smiling reads, *Welcome to Parenthood!* Two bottles,
a reusable nipple, and a tin of powdered baby formula are inside.
I let the packaging fall to my feet as I riffle through its contents
with morbid curiosity. My doctor's office must have given my
name to a formula company for advertising purposes, and it feels
like a betrayal. My name and address were likely added to a list
generated in mass, and packages would have been lined up on
factory assembly lines, waiting to be stamped with each name.
Nobody would have followed up to see if I actually had a baby
to feed. Nobody would have thought that targeting vulnerable
women—those who are pregnant or postpartum—could be a
harmful advertising tactic. Never mind how many would have
lost their baby to miscarriage or stillbirth.

I wonder how many other women like me received this package. If others are standing in the cold in another neighbourhood,
holding identical boxes in their hands, crying over this callous gift.

I walk back home, cradling the box, and I silently enter our
house. Joey is playing with Teddy in the living room, his voice
booming as they pretend to be dinosaurs. I tiptoe upstairs quietly,

the package still in my arms. I don't want Joey to see it. I place the box in my closet, tucking it behind the boxes of unused hormones and injections I stopped taking when I lost the baby. I no longer need these things, but I can't yet part with any of them.

Teddy and I are walking down the steps to our home after a playdate. Teddy's friend, who is also two, is about to become a big brother. His mom is going to have another boy in a matter of weeks.

"Who is my brother?" Teddy asks me, when we pause on our walk to pull some weeds from the garden.

"You don't have a brother," I reply gently, trying to hide the sadness in my voice. I know he is looking for answers and not pity.

"Are you my brother?" he asks, perhaps thinking the words *brother* and *mother*, which sound so alike, have a similar meaning.

"No, love. I'm your mother. Your mama." I hope that my reminding him who he has will make up for who he does not.

"I should get one," he says absentmindedly, while pulling at a dandelion. The head of the flower pops off and the green stem stands naked in the earth.

"Maybe someday," I reply, letting my voice trail off as we continue to the front door.

"Who's going to play with me?" Teddy asks in a high-pitched, tired voice. Tears spill from his almond-shaped eyes, tracking like rivers down his angry red cheeks.

I am trying to make supper and his hunger in the late afternoon often amplifies his sadness at being made to play alone. I think about my first miscarriage: two five-year-olds would have made great playmates for my son. I put on an audiobook, giving Teddy an apple, and I encourage him to play with his toys on his own. I promise to play with him again after supper.

I wonder if these first rumblings of loneliness, of a life without a sibling, are changing who my son will become. Are they creating a resilience? A natural tendency to play imaginatively and a solace in being alone? Or are they creating a co-dependence between mother and child, a need to have my presence occupy his days?

I try to balance fostering his independence with getting on the floor with him and playing in the world of his imagination. We are Transformers, dinosaurs, princesses twirling in our dresses. He likes to run and be tickled, silly word games, and making our own lyrics to songs as we go.

I am his mother, his playmate, and I cannot substitute for a missing sibling. But I am creating a void when, in his mind, there isn't one. I see my son as a sibling, but he is not. Joey and I are navigating foreign territory, trying to raise a child to not feel the loss of this even though we feel it acutely.

ONE MORNING, I SEE A CO-WORKER AT THE PLAYGROUND. We aren't overly familiar, but we know each other well enough to smile and nod in the hallways of the hospital. He doesn't see me. He is there with his wife and what appears to be family, or close friends. His daughter looks to be about four by the way she is roaming confidently around the playground. I look at him and his wife, scanning the periphery for the telltale signs of another child. A stroller with a sleeping baby, a toddler on a swing, an older child claiming to be bored. I see no evidence of a second child.

I wonder out loud to Joey, who is sitting on the bench beside me while Teddy tries to climb the metal slide, if he thinks their family is complete or if maybe their other child is on a playdate, or a grandparent is watching them. I can't help myself. I am constantly comparing and looking for a reflection of my family. I wonder what I am seeking in this comparison, the thief of joy. Am I scrutinizing each family to find other possible versions of myself? Or am I poking an old wound repeatedly until it opens up again?

My dreams fill in the gaps later on that night. I see my co-worker walking away from the playground holding hands with his four-year-old, an older child meeting them where the sidewalk begins. *Ah,* my voice in my dream says, *they're not like me after all.*

This involuntary reaction on the playground plays on a loop everywhere I go. I see parents with only one child and the absence of a sibling is as apparent as the child's existence. My son's life feels as tangible as my other babies' deaths. The undercurrent of my life is coloured with loss, like the trim in our house that I painted fresh white when we first moved in. The deep knots of the pine always break through, showing up like scars no matter how many coats I apply. We are a family built on contradictions. We are complete and incomplete, filled with deep pain and tremendous joy. Teddy is an only child who is not quite that.

25

▼

We told Teddy I was pregnant four days before we lost the baby. Our baby was fine at the moment, despite all our complications. It was beating its heart and growing bigger than expected for such a tiny little thing. All good signs, even for someone like me. And we had that ultrasound photo. Something tangible we cling to, when all the times before we had nothing to show for our lost babies.

At the time, we felt that telling our son was an act of inclusion. To tell him why Mama kept going to the doctor and what it meant to have a baby in my belly. Now that my belly was protruding, and it was occupying much of our conversation in front of our precocious child, we wanted him to hear it from us first. And so, we told him during supper one night.

He looked at me quizzically and asked, "You have a baby in your belly?" He was somewhat skeptical.

I mustered up the courage to say, "Yes, buddy. And they're going to grow and grow and grow and you will get to be a big brother." He didn't say much else after that. He finished his food and went to play with his toys.

In hindsight, it's easy to say that we were foolhardy. To tell a toddler, with only the most basic of understanding, that another baby was on the horizon. You could say we were reckless in telling our son because of our complicated past. But what I see, when looking back, are two people desperate for their baby to be real. By inviting our son into the conversation, we were believing this family into being. The last remaining sliver of hope that this child had to make it. This baby would now have to survive, because we had said so.

By wrapping our son around my pregnancy, in its desperate last days of existence, we thought we were protecting our future baby with the toughest, most precious thing we had. We were giving this child, the one in my tummy, the gift of our living son's acknowledgement. When we lost the baby, our son lost his sibling, the first one he knew about.

Days after my miscarriage, my son points at my belly and asks, "Mama, do you have a baby in your belly?"

"No, honey," I say gently. "No baby today."

He is a bit too young to ask many questions, but the next day he tries again.

"I'm going to be a big brother," he announces, while I am tying his shoes in the hallway.

"Actually, love," I say, "you're not going to be a big brother just yet."

He looks at me with question in his eyes, but he lets me off the hook. He is not yet of the age when he will ask me all the whys he feels in his heart.

I am grateful to not have to explain to him what my body has done. I want to protect him from the truth of who I am.

SOME DAYS I DON'T KNOW WHERE TO PUT MY GRIEF, SO I TAKE it with me, and I usually land in my bed. My tears leave permanent stains on my white pillowcase as I curl under the weight of my longed-for babies. "Who is it tonight?" I whisper to the darkness of my room. Sometimes it is my meant-to-be first-born twins, whom I imagine being bigger than my son is now. Hands that would still hold mine when we crossed the street, but children in beds instead of a toddler in a crib. Sometimes it is for the one whose due date is approaching. The baby whose head I was meant to smell while I would kiss their sweet neck as it lies close to my mouth. I can feel tiny fingers wrap themselves around mine and their weightlessness in my arms feels fragile, as if they could disappear at any moment. I long to care for my unborn children with the same vigilance I had for my newborn son, not allowing a moment to pass without counting their breaths. Even with them gone, I cannot let go of my need to keep them alive.

I never know exactly who it is I am missing because I never truly knew them. Can you miss somebody you've never met? Can you mourn a baby you never held? I often feel as if I have left something in another room, but when I turn to retrieve it, the room no longer exists. These babies are figments of my imagination, dates on a calendar that go unnoticed by anyone except me. They are stories I tell and scars I wear. They are me. An invisible, unbearable, significant part of me. And that's all they will ever be.

I thought grief had a beginning, middle, and an end. I didn't know it would be something I'd have to live with, in its ever-evolving form, forever. It belongs to me and I cannot separate myself from it. There are days it winds itself around my neck and others when I barely notice its presence. I feel it constantly, a companion I never wished for but one I have grown to love for what it represents. I couldn't hold the children I lost, but the grief I walk with is the tangible proof of their existence, even if I'm the only one who knows.

People want grief to be sad and pretty and for you to fold gently into their arms and accept whatever words they send your way. Grief is not pretty. It is angry and it is ugly. In those first few weeks after miscarrying, I am wild with grief-stricken rage. I snap and I snarl, Joey approaching me like I'm a tiger he wishes to tame. I look for things I can crush with my hands and I scream in my car until my voice grows hoarse. I sob deeply, until there is nothing left. Joey tiptoes through the house knowing what is happening inside is something he simply has to wait out.

I try to remember I won't always feel this way, but it's impossible to believe during those early days when your chest is tight and panic is your guide through the world.

One night, I change into my pajamas early. It is well before Teddy's bedtime. I throw my clothes on the chair in our bedroom that has never been sat in. I walk over to my side of the bed, turning on the dim lamp on my bedside table, and I curl up.

My phone is in my hand and I tell myself not to look. It never makes me feel better.

I ignore my own advice.

I open up the photos app and scroll back in time, past the photos of my son dressed in his new winter boots, jumping in a rain puddle, and the ones of him wearing his Halloween costume. I slow my scrolling when I reach our friends' wedding. I move my finger down the screen, swiping past the first dance, the ceremony, the selfie I took of the dress I wore, the subtle baby bulge. I go past the photos of the blue sky I took on our drive, my son napping in his car seat.

I pause, and swipe one last time.

There it is. The black and white thumbnail of a photo that makes my heart rate quicken. I click on it. The screen fills with the image that makes my throat tight. Our baby. I run my fingernail over their tiny nose, a little thigh. I place my finger over the hand that is waving playfully, trying to feel them through the screen. Had things gone differently, I would have printed this image, taping it inside a baby book with the label *Your first photo*. Tears pool on my pillow and I click off my phone. The photo is like a poultice for my grief, drawing out my sadness in metred doses.

I hear small footsteps on the stairs and the creak of the floorboard outside my door. The mattress bounces slightly, the springs squeaking beneath the weight of my son. I feel the weight of his body flop onto mine and his arms wrap around me, he becomes the big spoon.

"Mama, are you big sad?"

I pat his arm. "Yes, honey. Mama is big sad today."

"My hugs will make you better." He squeezes me tightly and I close my eyes, feeling the warmth of his breath against my cheek.

I HAVE OFTEN WONDERED IF MY BRAIN IS SOMEHOW BROKEN, just like my uterus, making these losses feel worse than they should. Or perhaps, like all of us, I have simply been conditioned into thinking a miscarriage does not claw at your insides for years after, leaving a permanent wound that can hurt without warning.

I have been told *These things happen, At least it happened early,* and *Thank goodness you have your son* so many times that I have begun uttering those same words out loud. Yet, I am always left unsatisfied with the comfort they are meant to bring.

When Joey and I travelled to New York City years earlier on our first miscarriage trip, I bought myself a necklace, a tiny bean on a delicate chain. It was a talisman of the first of my lost pregnancies. I wear my pain around my neck, like the grief that is often high in my throat. Over the years, I have gathered more. A necklace with a *T* for my son, and a simple *Mama* on a chain. I wear my necklaces as a reminder that I am a mother, was a mother, to all of them. The before, the after, and the in-between. I remind myself I loved them all so much. Even the ones I only carried for days. I loved them with a fervour that brought grief into my life forever.

I have discovered that grief is not something to endure in order to become un-bereaved. It is something you learn to live with, an unwanted companion that, at times, you scream at, and others, you cling to, because it's the only thing reminding you that what you lost was real.

26

▼

AT NIGHT, WHEN I CAN'T SLEEP, I FEEL THE PAIN OF GRIEF IN
each of my bones: scapula, sternum, tibia, fibula, femur. I place
my hand over each ache and name it out loud, whispering while
Joey sleeps beside me. I don't have names for my pregnancies, the
babies that would never be. They are numbered, given the most
basic of labels. Naming them won't make them any more real.

IN MY SECOND YEAR OF UNIVERSITY, DURING AN ANIMAL BIOLOGY
class, our lab instructor hands each pair of students the preserved
body of a cat we will dissect over the next several weeks. The
smell of formaldehyde permeates my white lab coat and clings
to the fabric of whatever clothes I wear underneath. No matter
how hard I wash them I can't seem to get rid of the vinegar-like
scent that stings my nostrils during those labs.

My lab partner, Mike, and I are handed a black tabby cat. I
don't think to ask where these cats came from; I'm here to act
the part of a serious biologist, and I'm focused on learning as
much as I can. I can't help my sadness, though, when I see her
pink toes and the pads of her paws. Her feet remind me of the
pet cats I grew up with and loved.

We dissect the abdomen first. I cut a tentative line along the
cat's belly with a sharpened scalpel, holding it awkwardly in a
gloved hand. Mike and I follow the instructions in our lab book
while our instructor paces the aisles, peering over shoulders,
pointing a finger at noteworthy organs.

She approaches our bench. Her grey hair is pulled back into
a low messy bun and she pushes her round, metal glasses up her
face with her forearm.

"Look here," she says, sticking an un-gloved finger into the cut we've made. "That's the uterus."

We glance at our open textbook, trying to see it the way she does, but bodies never look the same as they do in diagrams or figures. There are no colour-coded organs to decipher when you dissect a body. The red-purple of everything makes it hard for our beginners' eyes to see the organs clearly. Only the distinct yellow of fat tissue is easy to discern.

"Pull the uterus out," she instructs, and Mike complies, as though performing a hysterectomy. "Now, when you cut into the uterus, be careful. The wall is muscular, so it might be tough. Just take your time."

Mike picks up the scalpel this time and I hold the body of the cat steady while he performs a rudimentary C-section. Once the tissue gives way to a cavity beneath, we look at each other with wide eyes. When our cat died, she had been pregnant. Behind the wall of the uterus is the profile of a small kitten.

We call our instructor back and she says, "Yes, I thought that was the case. Normally, the uterus is not so swollen, but when pregnant, the cavity grows to accompany the fetuses inside. Well done." She leaves to answer another hand up in the air.

Mike and I look at each other hesitantly, unsure how to tackle our next task. He puts his fingers into the cavity and pulls out the kitten. He places it into my hands, and I receive the small creature as though he is handing me a newborn baby.

The kitten is wet, its bones not yet ossified, so its body feels as though it's full of thick liquid, like a sack of Jell-O not quite set. Mike reaches back into the uterus and delivers another kitten, and another. Five unborn kittens line the edge of our laboratory bench and we look disturbingly at our discovery. The instructor tells everyone to approach our bench. They gather around us, and she reviews the estimated gestation of the kittens based on their fused eyelids and absence of fur. She passes a kitten around for each student to feel in their hands, to understand the way in which bodies are formed through a series of cellular division and ossification of bone.

When everyone returns to their seats, the lab is nearly over. We are told to clean our areas and place our specimens in a plastic container for the following day. Our instructor tells Mike and I to put the kittens into the yellow biohazard bag she has placed in front of us. We are not going to dissect the kittens, and I am relieved we won't have to put a scalpel to their delicate skin.

Before cleaning up our area, I ask Mike, "Should we name them?"

Our instructor has told us not to name our animal cadavers. We are to treat them with respect and dignity, but naming them, she warns, might get in the way of science. We have already ignored her advice, having named our cat Whiskers.

"I don't think so," Mike says, though he sounds unsure. He is a kind-hearted person; he dreams of becoming a physician, but his squeamish nature will make it impossible. He will one day earn his PhD in mathematics, finding numbers and calculations more palatable to blood and guts. I know he is bothered by our discovery as well.

"Maybe we should give them numbers," he suggests, and I shrug my shoulders in response.

We place each kitten gently into the yellow bag, counting quietly to five, and then seal the top. We hand the bag to our instructor and she takes it to a large garbage bin down the hall marked *Caution: Biohazardous Waste*. I leave the lab somberly, remembering how the kittens felt in the palms of my hands. Even though we didn't name them, we write diligently about the fetuses in our lab report, numbering them and remarking on the unique characteristics of each. They didn't need names to be recorded and spoken about with such certainty. They existed anyway.

I'VE BEEN SEEING HEATHER FOR MONTHS WHEN SHE ASKS ME to write letters to my unborn babies. She tells me it's an exercise in letting go, that it might allow me to release some of my pain, to move forward. I no longer contest her requests, since I can feel a difference in myself with every passing week. It is nice to have dedicated time to mourn and to speak out loud what I'm feeling to someone other than Joey, since he is grieving too. At home, the words flow onto the page as if they've been waiting within me this whole time. My writing is fluid, filled with love and apologies, and I feel connected to them in a way I haven't before. Writing to them feels like the only act of mothering I can do.

I sit in Heather's office the following week, my lined notebook open on my lap, and I read the letters I wrote. I have many to read, so it takes up much of our time. When I am done, Heather doesn't say anything. I look at her black ballet flats and I focus on the way her pants slide up when she crosses her legs, exposing her bare ankles, anything to ignore the silence.

"Those were beautiful, Joanne," she says, after what feels like a monumental pause.

I have always craved praise, but I am uncomfortable when it comes in such a direct way. I long to hear people say good things about me, but I doubt the truth of it when it is spoken. I always assume people are simply being kind. I remember as a kid, when I brought home report cards filled with As, my parents told me how proud they were of me, but nothing felt as good as when, later that night, I overheard my mom on the phone telling my grandmother how well I had done. I remember opening my bedroom door wider, eager to hear her words of praise echoing down the hallway, and when the topic changed to something else, closing my door quietly, unable to stop smiling.

"Thanks," I mumble, briefly looking up from her shoes.

Heather uncrosses her legs, her pants falling back down, and she leans toward me. "Okay, now that you've read your letters, I'm going to ask you to do another exercise before our next session."

I lean in, mirroring her body language. My notebook is still open in my lap. I look down and I can see the ink has smudged on the page where my tears have fallen. I rub at it slightly, but only make it worse.

"I'm going to ask you to write a response to your letters," Heather says. "I want you to personify your babies and have them write back to you. Do you think you can do that for next week?" Heather looks at her watch, and I know our time is up. I grimace, unsure I can accomplish the task. I understand the concept, but it feels silly to write from the perspective of my babies, who were small enough to fit in the palm of my hand. How could I possibly know what they'd want to say? What if I got it wrong?

"I'll try," I say, shrugging my shoulders.

"That's all I ask," she says, smiling, and the shuffle of her papers makes me reach for my coat.

I procrastinate all week. I pull out my notebook many times during the day, but the task feels impossible, and I always tuck it back into the drawer of my desk, the page still blank.

Finally, the night before I am to see Heather again, I sit on my bed and look at the moon outside my bedroom window. I am overcome with emotion as I imagine where my babies might be now, trying to summon the voices I never got to hear. I picture them as stars in the sky, as the shimmer of moonlight across the ocean, and I feel my heart squeeze with the pain of losing them, of not knowing them. I close my eyes and I can feel their presence because parts of them are still inside me. Their cells, like those of Teddy's, passed into my bloodstream and live within me as well. If anyone would know what they'd want to say, it is me. I reach for my notebook and I write for an hour, guided by the moonlight, filling myself with their existence.

The next day, I read the letters to Heather. Once I am done, she asks me to repeat the first line.

"*We were never meant to live beyond the confines of your body, and we know how much you loved us,*" I read.

"You needed to hear that," Heather says. "That is what's going to release you, Joanne. Even when writing from the perspective of those babies, you are trying to relieve yourself of the guilt."

I nod my head slowly, trying to absorb what Heather has pointed out. Even though I wrote those words, I didn't know what I was trying to say. Heather remains silent while I wonder if I will ever be able to move forward, how I will ever release myself from the guilt. This time, while Heather waits patiently, I don't try to fight the quiet. Instead, I search for answers in the silence.

IN MY EARLY TWENTIES, I LOVED CELEBRITY GOSSIP. I SCOURED websites that showed photos of celebrities getting coffee and coming out of the gym. I logged onto the internet with a Dell desktop that took up a large corner of my dorm room and checked my bookmarked pages often. I scrolled through them, the noisy click of my mouse hitting *next* until I reached the last page. I read about Britney Spears and Lindsay Lohan, their personal traumas turned into household entertainment. When Heath Ledger died, I called my sister and we lamented the loss of a celebrity we both loved as I clicked through his photos.

And now, in the middle of a sleepless night, I reach for my phone on my bedside table. I search "celebrities who've had miscarriages" and I click on the first page. I read quotes and scroll through Instagram pages, as though looking for comfort from an old friend. I feel both twenty and thirty-two when I perform this late-night ritual of trying to feel less alone.

My Google search history reveals a lot about my insecurities. "How many miscarriages is a lot?" I ask the modern-day Magic 8-Ball. The results are inconclusive, akin to *Ask again later*. I click through online discussion boards instead, searching for women like me, hoping they exist somewhere.

One night, Joey and I watch a new show. It's part comedy, part dark drama, and my ears prick when it is revealed that a main character has had many miscarriages. My body tenses. I am leaning against Joey's chest, his arms wrapped around me in a hug. I wonder if he feels this too. The adrenaline-pumping desire to flee in response to a TV show. The feeling of cortisol rushing through your body, your deepest pain being dug up like a corpse.

I watch expectantly, anticipating the moment they reveal how many babies she's lost. I wonder if it will be more or less than me. I don't know what I am wishing for. I forget the plot, the dialogue becoming tinny, and my mouth goes dry.

The scene shifts. The woman is in the hallway of a hospital, her hands covering her face, while a doctor says, "I'm so sorry." My eyebrows crinkle and my lips form a straight line as I purse them together. I am building a dam out of muscles and skin.

The woman, now recounting that moment in the hallway, says, "That was my fifth one." I make a choking noise. Joey squeezes me tightly and I sob through the rest of the show, finally seeing myself on the screen. The woman receives sympathy from those to whom she tells the truth and I wonder if perhaps, someday, I will receive the same response. Maybe instead of asking Google for permission to grieve, I should have typed, "having miscarriages is a lot." And then turned off my phone.

I'VE STARTED TO DOCUMENT TEDDY'S PRESENCE WHEN HE ISN'T home. The books piled beside his crib. The rubber toys lining our bathtub. His shorts pulled off and hanging over the edge of the wicker hamper. They are shadows of his life, reminders that he is here. I oscillate between wanting to capture every moment on film and wishing to live each moment without a camera in hand, allowing his childhood to pass naturally. I could never fill enough clouds with videos and photos to allow me to relive the magic of his childhood. I simply have to live it.

Joey and I fill our walls with photos of our son at every age. Newborn, grinning toddler, all three of us together. We imprint our home with his existence. When I walk upstairs, I place my fingers against the nose of one-year-old Teddy grinning. Before I go to bed, I see a collage of NICU photos on my dresser, his feeding tube taped to the side of his cheek. He is everywhere.

Joey and I start to tell Teddy that our family of three is complete, even though I don't yet believe it myself. We simply don't want to encourage the desire for a sibling who may not appear. When we read a book about families, he says, "Mama, Dada, and Teddy," and I worry he feels hesitation when I repeat those words back. I wonder if he can intuit what I feel is lacking. We don't ask him if he would like a brother or a sister, feeling ourselves recoil when strangers bend down and utter those exact words. I know he would make a great sibling. I see it in the way he cares for Maddy, feeding her, petting her, and laughing at the way she rolls onto her back to itch a scratch. I see how gentle he is with our friends' babies. The way he shares his toys generously, laughing at them as though he is just another adult in the room.

I watch as his empathy for others bubbles over when we watch an emotional movie, his eyes filling with tears. I reach out and grab his hand when he is overcome with the emotion of a scene and he squeezes mine back in response. Joey and I look over his head at each other, smiling, unsure what to make of our child who feels so deeply, loving him even more for his tender care of others.

EVERY PARENT GIVES WOUNDS TO THEIR CHILD. AN UNINTENDED inheritance of pain is passed through cells and blood. My father, a Guyanese immigrant, lost his father when he was nine and moved to an unfamiliar country at eleven. The wounds of my father's childhood seep into my life through no fault of his. They persist in the absence of a grandfather, stories of a country I have only ever seen on a map, and how little is remembered, or spoken, of his early days in Canada. His life as a preteen was likely challenging. He was grieving the loss of his father and trying to learn the customs of a new place. We carry our wounds and pass them along to our children, linking each generation to the next like a chain of wilted daisies. Joey and I talk about what we have given Teddy, what pain he may hold because of us.

I am reading a book about motherhood when I stumble upon the term *mother's marks*. A term that was once used to describe the birthmarks or moles found on the bodies of babies and small children. It originated with the once-held belief that these imperfections on a child's skin were brought about by an ungratified longing in the mother.

I put my book down, feeling the weight of how much pressure women bear in carrying a child. We are told so many things will affect our unborn children. The way we sleep can impair blood flow in the umbilical cord, our emotions can change the heart rate of tiny fetuses, the things we put into our bodies will also go into theirs, causing potentially irreparable damage. No soft cheeses or uncured meats, no sushi, no cold medication, no stress, no overexertion. According to ancient lore, a mother must fulfill each of her heart's longings prior to conception, or forever risk marking her child.

I look at Teddy, who is playing on the floor nearby. When he stretches his arm to reach for a toy beyond his grasp, the sleeve of his shirt pulls up slightly, revealing his wrist. And I remember.

I sit on the floor beside him and I playfully tug off one sock. He giggles and asks, "What are you doing, Mama?"

I smile and say, "I want to see your foot." He lifts his leg compliantly, wiggling his toes, a pudgy foot proudly on display.

I hold his bare foot in my hand and place my thumb over the mole I've lovingly stroked since his infancy. It has grown with him, the once-tiny, barely noticeable speck now an obvious imperfection on his pale skin. I put his foot down and reach for his right arm, gently pushing up the sleeve of his light-blue shirt. I touch a second mole above his wrist. His two mother's marks. My two lost pregnancies before him. I kiss the top of his head and he smiles at me. Perhaps he is more marked by my grief than I realize.

27

▼

I am still mourning when I go to have a drink with a friend. I sip red wine on a comfortable couch, my legs tucked beneath me, clutching a pillow to my chest. I spend what feels like hours talking about my latest miscarriage. Grief makes me selfish. She listens intently, offering words of comfort and support. When I am done speaking, and finally ask her about her life, she casts her eyes downward.

"I have something to tell you," she starts, "but I'm scared to." She takes a sip of her wine.

"You can tell me anything," I urge her gently. I feel desperate to return the gift of listening she has just provided me.

"I had an abortion." She looks at me with a sadness in her eyes, not for herself, but for me. "I was so scared to tell you because I didn't want you to be upset. Here you are trying to have a baby and I am doing the opposite. I didn't want to make you feel worse."

I reach across the couch, putting my hand on her knee. "I'm so sorry. I totally get why you felt that way, though." I feel ashamed that she felt she couldn't turn to me. I feel like a bad friend, selfishly consumed with my own life, even though I understand her hesitation in telling me was an act of protection and love.

I ask for details. She walks me through when it happened—months earlier—with a man she barely knew. A man we had both known was bad news. They had been together briefly, and she had the procedure when she was five weeks pregnant, knowing it was the right thing to do. She tells me how she bled for days after and the cramps were hardest at night. I nod, asking if she had clutched a heating pad or taken naproxen to ease the pain.

Had she bled for weeks afterwards or was it over in days? We share the similarities of our stories, lamenting the invisible pain of women, and I discover the physical side of abortions is the same whether they are unwanted or chosen.

I ask her how she felt after. Emptied out, like me? Did she grieve in any way? She tells me she felt lighter, relieved even, knowing she made the right decision. Her pregnancy had not been wanted. A baby made by chance, a combination of luck, timing, and lack of contraception. I am intrigued by what she says, the way she describes it as an empowering choice.

I envy her power. The power to control what was happening inside her body, when I had no say in mine. I feel no judgment over her decision to end the pregnancy, but I am jealous that she got to choose what was best for her life. I feel myself stiffen, once again, with the lack of control I have over my body.

JOEY AND I ARE TUMBLING THROUGH THE WEEKS THAT FOLLOW our fifth miscarriage. Our grief has swallowed us, and we agree that we can't get pregnant again. Not now. We need time to heal. Jumping from one pregnancy to the next is doing nothing to ease our pain. Moving forward this time means pausing. Breathing. Allowing ourselves to feel everything. We want to try and heal properly without a new pregnancy interrupting the process.

In the weeks that follow a miscarriage, I take pregnancy tests to monitor my hormone levels. With every passing day, the lines grow fainter until the test finally declares that I am not pregnant. I run out of pregnancy tests weeks after I miscarry this time, and instead of buying more, I use the ovulation tests I still have in my bathroom cupboard. I know that these tests can act as a poor man's pregnancy test, as ovulation and pregnancy hormones are so similar. No doctor would advise me to use them in this way because the results can be confusing. But I use them anyway, and wait until it displays a single line, indicating a total absence of pregnancy hormone. The following day, the lines brighten up again, looking just like the positive ovulation test displayed on the box. I think for a moment that perhaps the test means I am ovulating, but I toss it into the garbage, not allowing the seed of a thought to take root.

That night, Joey and I make love. A desperation has grown between us, a desire to feel joy and find safety in the familiarity of each other's embrace. The morning after, I check the calendar and think about the bright ovulation test I had tossed aside the day earlier. I calculate the weeks since my surgery—four—and the likelihood that the test means I am ovulating. The seed that took root the day before has bloomed and I rip open another ovulation test, the purple packaging tearing apart in my trembling hands. After waiting two minutes, I glance at the test.

"Shit," I say out loud. The lines are faint again, meaning the previous day's test had likely picked up a surge in ovulation hormone and was not reflective of my past pregnancy. It meant I was ovulating when we had sex.

It is Thanksgiving weekend and we are driving to visit Joey's parents when I blurt it out.

"I took an ovulation test yesterday," I start, glancing at Joey whose eyes are fixed on the road. "It was positive, and I think it meant I was actually ovulating." I feel shame course through my body. Joey glances over at me and anger flashes across his face. I look down.

"Jo," he says, his fear coming at me like anger. "Why wouldn't you tell me this before? Do you really want to be pregnant right now? Because I can't handle that."

His hands grip the steering wheel and I look down at my lap. His accusation makes me question what I have done. What was I thinking? Did I secretly want to get pregnant even though a new pregnancy would break me? I feel as though I was careless with myself, reckless with our marriage.

Joey seethes, assuming the worst of me in those moments. He knows my inclination has typically been to get pregnant as quickly as possible after a miscarriage. I use the hope for a new pregnancy as a way to focus on the future, to blunt the pain of the present. He has grown tired of that cycle. He is exhausted from bearing the brunt of my grief and he needs time to consider what he wants. He feels as though I have left him out of the equation. He feels tricked, as though I am lying.

I try to explain to Joey that I didn't try to trick him. But even I doubt the truth of that; my own explanations sound like lies I am telling myself. Maybe I am doing what I always do, making big decisions on my own and expecting Joey to follow. He is angry the rest of the drive and my claims feel dishonest, even to me, my words falling flat, as though too heavy to be carried through the air. My insistence feels panicked, my excuses weak. I feel like a child, being punished for something when I don't have the words to explain what I have done.

We arrive at my in-laws barely speaking. I am remote during Thanksgiving dinner. I try to follow the conversation, but I begin to fear another pregnancy with the same intensity I assume Joey is feeling. When we retreat to bed later that night, I roll over to my husband, whose back is turned away from me, and I put my arms around him. He rolls over and pulls me close.

"I'm sorry," he whispers into my ear. He has always been better at forgiveness than me.

"No, I'm sorry. I don't know why I didn't think about it until after," I say honestly. "Maybe a part of me was doing what I always do and really wanted to be pregnant again. Maybe I'm not capable of making rational decisions right now. I'm just really sad." I cry softly, and he cups his hand against my cheek, his thumb wiping my tears as they fall.

"I know," he says gently. "I'm really sad, too."

I tell him I have a plan to solve our problem. I will go to the pharmacy the next day and take the morning-after pill. I still have time, since you can take the pill up to seventy-two hours after having sex. The next morning will mark thirty-six.

We make an excuse the following morning to make a quick stop at the store. I run into the pharmacy, feeling a sense of duty, a sense of control. I ask the pharmacy assistant for the morning-after pill. She is younger than I am, and she tells me it is on the shelf behind me, but she will grab one from out back, saving her time later when she has to restock the shelves.

"Do you want to speak with the pharmacist?" she asks, ringing in my purchase.

"No," I reply. "I'm good."

I buy the single pill, encased in a white and purple box. I wonder if purple was chosen to reflect the blending of pink and blue. Or perhaps they chose a colour that doesn't remind people of baby blankets and soft toys, the deep purple darker than the shades babies tend to be surrounded by.

When we return to Joey's childhood home, I go into the bathroom, pulling out the contents of the box, laying them neatly on the counter in front of me. The pill looks small, solitary. I open the plastic, releasing the white pill from its cell, and I hold it in my hand. I feel powerful. The smooth, rounded edge looks unassuming, but it feels menacing in my fingers. It has the ability to destroy. To evacuate my womb, preventing anything from taking hold. I breathe in through my nose and out through my mouth, telling myself I cannot get pregnant right now, that I want to take this pill.

I place the pill on the palm of my hand and tip it into my mouth, watching myself in the mirror. My hand stays covering my mouth for a moment and it looks like I am stifling a silent scream. I swallow the round pill down without water, gulping twice, feeling the pill make its way down my throat. When I feel it pass into the upper part of my stomach, I turn on the water and drink directly from the faucet.

I stand, wiping my wet mouth with the back of my hand, and place my other hand over my stomach. I feel no sadness; I feel empowered. I will the little pill to do its deed. To shed the lining of my uterus, to prevent a pregnancy that would further complicate my compound grief. I walk back to where Joey is waiting in the bedroom. I nod to him, sitting down beside him on the bed. We speak in hushed tones about how other people would not understand what had just transpired. How two people so desperate for another child would choose to end the hopes for a new pregnancy. He puts his arm around me, kissing the top of my head, and breathes a sigh of relief into my hair.

Later that night, I begin to feel cramps. I inhale the pain, allowing myself to absorb the reality of what they mean. For the first time in recent years, I have taken control of my fertility. I am a woman who is finally in charge of her fate.

As the first drops of blood hit my underwear, I retreat to the bedroom to grab a pad from my bag. For once I don't fear the blood. I have asked for it, begged it to come. As I ball up my bloody underwear, tucking it neatly in the bottom of my suitcase next to the empty pill box, I don't think about the baby that could have been. I think of the family that was. That is. My husband, my son, me. I think about how I would have been a shadow of myself had I become pregnant again so soon after my fifth loss. How it would have split me apart, breaking me into hundreds of pieces, and parts of me would have been lost forever. I think about how I have finally done the one thing that has been missing in all my years of trying to have children: I made a decision over the fate of a hypothetical child.

I go to sleep without trouble that night, even though the cramps rippling over my abdomen remind me of times past. They are welcome guests this time, not thieves who stole into my body uninvited. I imagine the scraping of my uterus as it pulses and radiates pain around my back, and for once, I don't feel the urge to apologize.

28

▼

My hair falls out. Big clumps of dark brown hair fill the drain and I hold handfuls of it after brushing my tender scalp, looking for bald spots in my bathroom mirror. Ulcers fill my stomach and my mouth is overtaken by thrush, making talking and eating almost unbearable. I break out in a full-body rash, sores appearing on the surface of my skin, popping in painful eruptions that seem to have no known source—I imagine the pain I am feeling inside is trying to escape. I develop a uterine infection and ovarian abscesses, my body handing out punishment after punishment reminding me of its heartlessness. Mine is not a body to be trusted.

I dream of running away. Not from my family or my life, but from a body that feels broken and a mind that pumps out anxiety like radiation from Chernobyl; a poisonous, invisible substance bent on my future destruction. I wonder what it would be like to have a body deliver a baby safely, on time, and without complication. How would it feel to be relaxed and sure of my body's ability to bear children?

To make the decision to get pregnant again feels like the heaviest of all. To pull the pin of a grenade and hold onto it, hoping it won't go off. To play Russian roulette with a loaded handgun. I don't want to explode my family. I don't want to destroy the happiness and love we have.

"It seems to me that you have a happy life," my doctor says to me. "And I know you can understand all the repercussions of these possibilities."

He has outlined all of the ways in which a future pregnancy could go badly. I have less than a twenty percent chance of carrying a baby to term. I am more likely to miscarry or to have a severely premature baby. Choosing to become pregnant feels like choosing death. Death of another embryo or fetus. Death of a child born too prematurely or incompatible with life. Death of my family. My sanity. My marriage.

How do I walk with the guilt I will forever have over pulling that trigger? Who am I to make such a careless decision about the lives of four people?

I am being selfish, I know that. And yet, I feel incomplete, and I don't know if the child-sized hole in my heart will ever be filled. I feel like a terrible mother for even considering getting pregnant again. I am still trying to learn how to care for the child in my arms while mourning the ones I will never get to hold. I am trying to balance the grief I have for the children who will never be, with the complexities of parenting a toddler. Some days I am better at mourning than I am at being patient with my son. Other days I discover I have gone two whole hours without thinking of my lost babies. And then a pregnant woman or a song or a date on the calendar will pull me out of my forgetting and I will grieve them all over again. It's the love turned grief that I have in my heart, reminding me I was their mother. Those tiny beans of a baby, the ones whose beating hearts were the size of a pen-tip.

I am trying to honour all of my would-be children. To make note of dates that were important, that are important. To remember how old they would be if only they had survived. They will never run into my arms or smile proudly and say, "I did it, Mama!" when they put their shoes on for the first time. They are frozen between life and death for eternity. They never got to live, so did they even die? When do we consider a life a life? I believe in a woman's right to choose and their right to say *not this baby, not this time, not for me*. But I also believe that the love I had for those tiny hints of life was as strong as if they were fully formed humans. My intimate knowledge of the human body does nothing to soothe my mind. I remind myself that an eight-week embryo is just a clump of cells. I tell myself how often miscarriages happen. I say out loud, "At least I have my son." None of these things bring the comfort they are meant to provide when I am mourning the loss of another life.

We love pregnancy in our society, but only one kind. We love the kind that doesn't appear until twelve weeks and shows a loving, heterosexual, able-bodied couple holding an ultrasound picture. We want to laugh at cravings (*Pickles! Ice cream!*), and the only complication we are comfortable with is mild morning sickness. We want babies to be born naturally, which is to say vaginally, and we want them to come out a healthy 7 pounds 4 ounces. We don't want to hear about miscarriages or bleeding, or markers on ultrasounds that could mean possible genetic conditions. We don't want to hear about all the ways in which things can go wrong, because it will upset our view of women. Women are meant to be fertile. We are meant to nurture life, to create it. To mother. If we examine the ways in which pregnancies can go badly, we upset the way in which women are meant to exist in this world.

Where does my desire to have children come from? Was it born from the Cabbage Patch Kid doll I used to carry as a child? A bald-headed infant with a beanbag body and a plastic head that smelled like strawberries. Maybe it's from the television I grew up watching in the nineties. The hyper-gendered world of nuclear families and children who looked like steps on a staircase when lined up. Or is there something biological inside that made me long for a child of my own? A natural tendency of womanhood to birth a child into reality. I can't untangle that web, and neither can Heather. Is my desire internal or is it culturally driven? Innate or due to my socialization? Does it even matter?

I wonder what it must be like to feel content. To feel whole, and that your family is complete. I wonder how it must feel to not carry the weight of shame and guilt over losing so many babies for so many years. To be pregnant, and certain with your future. I wonder what it might be like to let go of all of the should-haves and could-have-beens, and to accept this as my fate. To let go of who I thought I was for my entire life and to accept who I am. To walk away from the six years of turmoil this has brought into our lives and to live happily, without ticking fertility clocks sounding their alarms from the next room, without the fear that comes with a positive pregnancy test, and the anticipation of it.

I contemplate when and how I will tell our son about my miscarriages. I dread the moment he might ask for a sibling, and I wonder what he will think about his mother whose body failed her so miserably. I am unsure how he will feel that he was the one who made it. *The one who lived.* It is such a dramatic title, and yet I can't deny its truth. My hope is that he understands all the complexities of his conception and arrival into this world, and he does not feel a burden to represent a tiny army of lost babies. He is perfectly imperfect, and he owes the world, and his parents, nothing to make up for the mess my body has made of our family.

He shared a womb with the ghosts of babies who may roam the halls of our house. The complications of his pregnancy mirror those of my miscarriages and I cannot explain why he is here and they are not. I do not understand either the miracle of his survival or the pain of their loss. I don't know why so many babies died and only one survived. I do not yet know how to explain to my beautiful boy all the ways the world can both delight and harm you.

I worry about being a mother to an only child. I've heard utterances of the "selfish only child" on more than one occasion. My son may be an only child, or perhaps he will not. This will not determine whether or not he has a generous heart. He is sensitive and sweet in the most tender of ways that little boys can be. He is quick to share, quiet when overwhelmed, and proud when he tackles a new skill. My job, as his mother, is to foster his strengths as much as I possibly can. I will not resign myself to believing that should my body fail to produce another child, he is doomed to a life of selfishness. He will value his close friendships with our friends who have similarly aged children, and he will grow up alongside animals he can share his deepest secrets with. When he feels alone, I hope he reaches for the many books on his bookshelves so that he can realize that none of us is truly alone.

I want my son to look up to me, not to carry the burden of his six unborn siblings. I do not want him to grow up with a mother who is more concerned with what she doesn't have than grateful for what she has.

I sometimes imagine there is a version of me in the world who never lost a single baby. That I delivered my twins, and perhaps even went on to have another child. I wonder how that version of me is doing. Has she ever cried so hard that she burst the blood vessels in her eyes? Does she love her babies with the same intensity as I love my son? I am sometimes envious of this fictional version of myself, but I am wary of her hypothetical existence, because to erase the sorrow would be to also erase my son. It is not something I can wish for, because to have the pain is to also have him.

29

▼

I AM HAVING COFFEE WITH A CO-WORKER AND WE ARE TALKING about a woman whose infant tragically died at birth. A stillbirth. She detailed her experience in a beautiful essay and we were both moved when we read it, which lead to a discussion about the pain so many mothers bear.

"I would way rather have a miscarriage than a stillbirth," my co-worker tells me, pouring milk into her coffee. We are at a popular café, sitting at a wooden table, a small vase of pink carnations between us. Her spoon clinks inside the mug as the black coffee turns the colour of the oak table beneath it.

I wonder if she knows my history, and I decide that she must not, since she has so casually tossed these hurtful words my way. I smile and reassure her that I, too, would choose a miscarriage in that scenario of awful selections. I would also choose no miscarriages over five. We aren't given the choice of when or how our lives may career off the path we have envisioned for ourselves.

It has been five months since my last miscarriage. There are days I look at the scars on my stomach or notice my ever-looming would-be due date and I wonder, when did I become this woman? A woman who knows such sadness.

The days when I am struck by grief are becoming fewer and the way in which I need to accommodate my heartache is becoming less intrusive as the months wane. Time does not heal all, but the intensity of grief, the way you feel like your world has completely tipped on its axis, lessens. I am learning to live alongside my pain, trying hard to accept the woman I am today. I know I could have always suffered more, as my co-worker so eloquently pointed out, but that doesn't mean I have lost my right to feeling sad.

I understand how lucky I am. I have my son. I know how easily I could have lost him during my pregnancy or after delivery. I could have no children, and this story would be filled with a completely different type of pain. I understand all of this, and yet, I am still sad about the pregnancies I lost. Why can't I be both grateful and sad? Why do I need to prove my pain is worthy because what I lost is, quite literally, so small?

I am grateful and I am also sad. I don't think one cancels the other, they co-exist like two sides of a coin. I have been told to appreciate my life (I do) and to be grateful for my son (I am) but very few people have told me to feel sad, to let it seep into my veins and to feel it all. Sadness, for most, is not meant to be felt. It is meant to be survived, kept hidden from view, pushed away. I am incapable of doing any of that simply because I know no other way. Perhaps we need to re-imagine what it means to grieve. That if we, humans, are capable of such sadness, then sadness is inherently a part of being human. We are unprepared for it when it comes into our lives uninvited, and we are uncomfortable when we see it in others.

I feel immense joy for my son, and I also feel deep sorrow for the babies I lost. I don't need well-intended friends to tell me how great my life is, as though you can distract a person out of their grief. And even though I am sad, it does not mean I am not enjoying my son. I feel the joys of motherhood perhaps an octave higher than most. I understand how close I was to losing him, and there are very few days I forget the miracle that is his survival. It is why I refuse to mourn the loss of his babyhood. When older strangers look down at my toddler and say, "They grow up too fast. You'll long for these days again," I smile and nod, but in my heart, I am grateful he is growing. His growth is a gift. Having a toddler instead of a baby is like having a baby instead of a miscarriage. An inexplicable coordination of miraculous events had to happen perfectly in order for him to be here, and they did.

WE HAVE A LOT OF WORK TO DO IN SOCIETY FOR WOMEN LIKE me. We need places to go that aren't emergency rooms filled with callous doctors and unfeeling words. We need answers to all of the questions we have and, if I can be so bold, solutions to how we might stop a miscarriage from happening. I want a place that is caring and understands the complex emotions early pregnancy loss can produce. I don't wish for platitudes; I simply wish for care.

We also need to re-examine why we hide our pregnancies for so many weeks. What this does to the women who miscarry. We are receiving the message that our pregnancies did not matter. I do not wish to stand on the shoulders of pro-life activists, because I understand how everyone's experience is different. I would simply like to mourn my losses without feeling as though I am disrupting an entire social norm in the process. In my loftiest of dreams, I will one day open a centre for women like me. A place for women to receive answers by way of ultrasounds and tests, but also a place filled with empathy, where all staff will receive explicit instruction to never begin a sentence with the words *At least*.

People ask me how Joey has handled all of this. Most care about him deeply, and some are simply curious. Men are often left out of stories like mine, and Joey has his own version to tell. We hold different perspectives of a shared experience, and although for years I wished he would feel the same way as me, I have come to appreciate that we are two people simply trying to survive.

Joey has the luxury of not experiencing a miscarriage physically. He does not have to fear the blood and the pain, or deal with hormones that send him into a blind rage. I, however, don't know what it's like to lose a spouse to grief for weeks and months at a time. He has to pick up the pieces of my broken heart that I strew about our house like dirty laundry. He walks around in those early days after a miscarriage holding everything together, waiting for the moment I return.

Joey kisses my head each time I walk into the OR to undergo another D and C. Before the double doors between us close—the ones that have the words *Do Not Enter. Restricted Access* etched in red on their windowless exterior—he tells me how proud he is of me. I am usually being escorted down a long, cold corridor by a nurse, shuffling in my socked feet, my IV acting like a too-short leash between us. Knowing Joey is behind me, sitting in that cramped waiting room, gives me the courage I need to keep walking. He is the one waiting, trying not to glance at the clock too often, wondering why one surgery is taking twenty minutes longer than the last. When I wake, and I am in my anesthetized stupor, I can still feel his hand holding mine.

Joey was there when Teddy was born, watching while I was jostled around the table like a ragdoll as the surgeon tugged and pulled him out. He, too, was fearful of our son's untimely arrival, but he never admitted how scared he was. He was encouraging and supportive, whispering words of positivity into my ear and squeezing my hand when I received my epidural. The day after Teddy was born, in a voice filled with emotion, Joey turned to me and said, "I can't believe what you did for us, Jo. What you did for me." His eyes held such love and admiration that even as I stood in front of him in my mesh underwear, my stomach still swollen, milk leaking from my breasts, I had never felt more beautiful.

Joey is the only one who understands the complex feelings another pregnancy would bring because he feels them too. He has worn the brunt of my anger and he has handled each loss with an optimism I lost along the way and am trying to regain. He encourages me to write, to sleep in, to tell him everything I am feeling, without asking for much in return. We speak about the future, about all of the what-ifs, and the only thing we are certain of is each other. We don't know if we will allow ourselves to hope for more children, the dream we have held onto for so long, or if we will move forward with our happy family of three. We have decided adoption is not the decision for us right now, and if we are to change our minds about this, I know better than to let grief lead the way. These are big decisions that feel heavy and grim, but knowing we are making the choice together allows me to believe we will be okay.

Joey worries about my mental well-being, about how much grief I can handle. He pushed me, gently, to talk about our story—my version of it—in a way that might allow me to move forward. He was the one who encouraged me to talk to someone and, on the morning I first left for Heather's office in the middle of winter, who hugged me and said, "I'm so proud of you, Jo, for getting help. But please, don't try to be good at therapy. Just go and do it."

I learned a lot during my time sitting on Heather's blue couch. How our minds deceive us and how women, and mothers, are held to impossibly high standards, most often by ourselves. I spoke negatively to myself for many years, and it is taking a lot of work to unravel the damage I have unknowingly caused. I am still working to release myself from the guilt before its roots grow too deep, and I am learning to take myself by the hand, repeating four words like a mantra, *This isn't your fault.*

My life as a mother who has dealt with loss means I cannot always be objective about Teddy's well-being. I am always on the alert for signs he is ill or hurt. Joey and I will ask each other, "Does he look pale to you? Does he seem quieter today? Do you think he's all right?" This feels like a failure as a nurse, my well-trained brain unable to drown out my fears, but I cannot keep back the thoughts that something might take him from me. My love for him, though, does not need to be forever entwined with my fear for his life. They can become untangled; they are becoming unwound.

My hope for my son is that he is learning how to handle the challenges that life can bring by watching his mother. Teddy has seen me go through the emotions of loss without understanding the complexities of grief. My fear is that he will be deeply affected if I am unable to relinquish the guilt and shame I have carried. That if I am unable to resolve the effects of trauma within myself, he will inherit the parts of my story I do not wish to pass along. I am working on releasing myself, so that he may be released as well.

The sad days still come, and I am learning how to give grief the space it needs in my life to breathe. I will sneak away from my desk at work for a moment, locking the bathroom door, and cry for a few minutes alone. I look at that ultrasound photo more often than I care to admit. As I write this, the due date of my last baby is fast approaching. Those days are always heavy. My eyes will burn, and I will go to bed early, curling under the covers, longing for a baby to hold.

Before having Teddy, I thought a baby would erase all of the grief I felt for the miscarriages I had. I believed my infertile self would die the moment a baby of mine survived, that a baby was the only thing separating me from the before and after versions of myself. I assumed becoming a mother would forever disconnect me from the infertile woman I once was because my longing for motherhood had felt unbearable. Even as I write this, allowing myself to fall back into the space of grief and longing for motherhood, I feel a twinge of jealousy for the woman I am now. I am her reflection, her fertile twin. I have crossed over to the other side of longing and am now firmly rooted in motherhood.

Since having my son, I've realized I will never become the happy "after" photo I assumed I would be. I am the space between motherhood and longing for it, but it's a space that doesn't exist. I can't be both fertile and infertile; our language doesn't allow for it. So, this is the space I have created for myself. This is where I live. Forever fertile and infertile. A mother to six, a mother of one. I am childless, and with child. Barren and fruitful. Pregnant and then not. Lucky, unlucky.

There will come a day when I no longer carry spare clothes and wipes in my oversized purse for Teddy. When I don't fill my pockets with toys and snacks to distract a small toddler. As I shed the largeness of early motherhood—diapers, strollers and car seats—like layers shed on a warm autumn day, I will still be a mother. Whether I have another child or not, whether I lose another child or not, I will still be a mother. I am his mother.

Epilogue

▼

TEDDY IS THREE WHEN JOEY AND I DECIDE WE WANT TO TELL him. To have the story of our family's creation be something he always knew. We don't want our son to have the memory of us sitting him down one day, saying, "We have something to tell you."

We planned to tell him after a summer holiday with our friends, one of whom is eight months pregnant. We thought we'd casually start up a conversation with Teddy on the drive home about babies and subtly mention how sometimes, babies don't grow. We planned the moment vaguely, thinking the words would come when the moment was right.

We don't get to enact our plan.

One afternoon, while Teddy is looking through a book about two male penguins who become parents, he looks at me and asks, "Why wasn't the baby there before?" He points to the part in the book when the baby penguin hatches from her egg and the two fathers are looking at her proudly.

"She wasn't born yet," I reply, sitting up straighter in my chair, facing him. "You have to be born and then you get to live." My nerves tingle with the foreshadowing of where this conversation may be heading. It is a sunny July afternoon and we have taken our books outside to read together. We are sitting on our back deck, listening to the light wind rustle the leaves around us and the faint crash of the ocean nearby.

"Where was I before I was born?" Teddy asks, crinkling his eyebrows together.

"You were a wish. We didn't have a baby before you." My heart beats a little faster and I feel the familiar lump forming in my throat, anticipating what he is about to ask next.

"Why didn't you have a baby before me?"

When you're three, the world is full of whys. Why are some people big and some people small? Why do we have fingernails? Why do you say you love me? Why?

I wonder if I will lack the courage to tell him.

"Well," I start, pausing to keep my voice steady, "Mama once had six other babies in her belly, but they couldn't grow big enough to be born." I show him with my fingers how small babies are when they are first conceived, holding my thumb and forefinger closely together.

"Babies start out as tiny specks," I explain, "and then they grow, and grow, and grow." With my hands, I mime my stomach becoming larger. "Then, the mama's belly gets as big as a watermelon!"

Teddy giggles at the image and I reach out to tickle him.

"When you were born," I say, turning more serious as I place my hands on his knees, "you were our first baby who was able to grow into being born. And now you are a big boy."

He smiles. He loves being called a big boy.

"Mama's other babies stayed really small." I lift my right hand and, with my fingers outstretched, I slowly bring my fingers and thumb closer together, until my forefinger and thumb look as though they are holding an invisible blueberry. "My other babies didn't get to grow, so they never got to be born, like you." I finish my explanation by placing the palm of my hand flat against my stomach.

"Why don't some babies grow?" Teddy asks.

"We don't always know, love. Some babies just don't." I don't feel sad admitting this; instead, I feel my anxiety abate, satisfied that I have finally told him my secret.

"I see," he says, turning back to his book about penguins. I look at his head bent over the book; his brown hair is curled tightly against his scalp in the intense summer humidity. His hair is damp, as he's just woken from a sweaty, mid-afternoon nap, and I can smell the sunscreen I rubbed into his soft skin hours ago.

I wonder if he feels the gravity of what I've just told him, if he is thinking about my other babies while he looks at the picture of the penguin cracking out of her shell, triumphant smiles painted on her parents' faces. Perhaps by telling him, the gravity of my admission has lifted. As though I've released a pressure valve I've held closed tightly for years, the air escaping with a high-pitched hiss. A contented silence follows.

I sit back in my chair and I tilt my head upwards, feeling the warmth from the sun on my face. I am awash with relief that he finally knows. I turn back to my book and Teddy is flipping through the pages of his quietly. The back door opens and we both look up. Joey steps out onto our wooden deck, squeezing into the chair beside Teddy. Joey's hair is turning grey, the scruff on his face speckled with white and silver. His smile is the same.

"Everything okay?" Joey asks. He puts his arm around Teddy's shoulders and his knee touches mine. The three of us are connected like a triangle, the strongest shape there is.

"Everything's okay," I say, and I feel lighter than I have in a long time.

Acknowledgements

▼

Thank you to everyone at Nimbus Publishing for your belief in this story and thinking it worthy enough to share with others.

To the Writers' Federation of Nova Scotia, thank you for the gift of the Alistair MacLeod Mentorship Program and for your endless support of writers like me. Carole Glasser Langille, my mentor and very first reader, thank you for your guidance, your friendship, and your generous words that encouraged me while working on the earliest version of this book.

Whitney Moran, my dear friend and editor, this would not have become a book without you. Your friendship, love, and care of me during my darkest hours helped me survive my hardest days. Your expertise, support, and encouragement allowed me to write and publish this book. *Thank you* will never be enough.

To the women I love dearly who have their own versions of this story to tell—Kellie, Kailee, Lisa, Jen, and Jenny—this is as much for you as it is for me. To all of my other friends and family who are too numerous to mention, I hope you know how supported and loved I have always felt by you.

Joey, thank you for encouraging me to write this story and for understanding how important it was for me to send it out into the world. Thank you for reading it and providing your input; it is infinitely better because of you. For your unconditional love and care of me during the most challenging times of our lives, I am forever grateful. I love you.

Teddy, my sweet, curly haired, beautiful boy. I wrote this for you, so that I could heal and be the type of mother you deserve to have. One day you might read this, and I hope you know how much I have always loved you. I love you more than all the stars in the sky, all the trees in the forest, and all the water in the sea. I am so glad you are here.

Recommended Reading

▼

Many of the following books helped inform and inspire me while writing this book. They provided me with guidance that I could not have found elsewhere, and they gave me the comfort of never feeling alone in my grief. Perhaps they will provide you some comfort as well.

Memoir

An Exact Replica of a Figment of My Imagination by Elizabeth McCracken
Blue Nights by Joan Didion
I Am I Am I Am by Maggie O'Farrell
I Had A Miscarriage by Jessica Zucker
Inferno: A Memoir of Motherhood and Madness by Catherine Cho
Notes for the Everlost: A Field Guide to Grief by Kate Inglis
Once More We Saw Stars by Jayson Greene
Shadow Child by Beth Powning
The Bright Hour by Nina Riggs
The Unwinding of the Miracle by Julie Yip-Williams
The Year of Magical Thinking by Joan Didion
This Is Happy by Camilla Gibb
Wave by Sonali Deraniyagala
When Breath Becomes Air by Paul Kalanthi

Non-Fiction

Mother is a Verb by Sarah Knott
The Seed by Alexandra Kimball
What God is Honored Here? edited by Shannon Gibbey and Kalia Yang

Fiction

Hamnet and Judith by Maggie O'Farrell
The Light Between Oceans by M. L. Stedman
The Birth House by Ami McKay
The Sea Captain's Wife by Beth Powning
Worry by Jessica Westhead

Graphic Novels & Picture Books

I Used to Have a Plan by Alessandra Olanow
Kid Gloves by Lucy Knisley
Rosalie Lightning by Tom Hart
The Heart and the Bottle by Oliver Jeffers
Wildflower by Briana Corr Scott